Don't
Go To The
Cosmetics Counter
Without Me

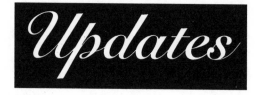

Newsletter

If you are interested in receiving subscription information about Paula Begoun's *Cosmetic Counter Newsletter* updates, available in June of 1992, just write to Beginning Press and we will send you the information as soon as it is available.

Updates

Beginning Press • 5418 South Brandon • Seattle, WA 98118

Don't Go To The Cosmetics Counter Without Me

An Eye Opening Guide To Brand Name Cosmetics

Paula Begoun

BEGINNING PRESS

Other books by Paula Begoun, available
by mail order from Beginning Press

Consumer:

Blue Eyeshadow Should Still Be Illegal . . . . $ 9.95

Travel:

The Best Places To Kiss In Northern California 9.95
The Best Places To Kiss In Southern California 9.95
The Best Places To Kiss In The Northwest 10.95
The Best Places To Kiss In New York City 10.95

To order any or all of these titles please send a check for the total
price of each book, plus $1.50 for shipping and handling to:

Beginning Press
5418 So. Brandon
Seattle, Washington 98118

Editors: Sheree Bykofsky, Carina Langstraat, Stephanie Bell
Art Direction: Steve Herold
Cover Design: Robert Pawlak
Typography: Lasergraphics
Printed in the United States by: R.R. Donnelley & Sons Company
                                  Harrisonburg, Virginia

Research Assistance: Carina Langstraat
© Copyright 1991 Paula Begoun
Publisher: Beginning Press
            5418 So. Brandon
            Seattle, Washington 98118

First Edition: June 1991
ISBN 1-877988-01-4
    4 5 6 7 8 9 10

This book is distributed to the United States book trade by:
      Publishers Group West
      4065 Hollis Street
      Emeryville, California 94608
      (415) 658-3453

and to the Canadian book trade by:
      Raincoast Books Limited
      112 East 3rd Avenue
      Vancouver, B.C., CANADA V5T 1C8
      (604) 873-6581

Dedication

This book is dedicated to the women in my life who understand the fun and frustration of striving to be the best they can possibly be in this world. Besides being wonderful people, none of them ever takes this beauty stuff too seriously, which is probably why they are the most attractive and remarkable women I know. Plus: they rarely go shopping for makeup without talking to me first. Trust and mutual respect are what make friendship so glorious.

Professional Acknowledgment

I would like to thank all the saleswomen I met who told me their true feelings and opinions about the cosmetics lines they were selling. I can't thank them by name because I would not want to jeopardize their jobs or careers, but their help was an invaluable tool in compiling the honest, no-holds-barred evaluations that made this guide possible.

Table of Contents

Publisher's Note

The intent of this book is to present the author's ideas and perceptions about the marketing, selling and use of cosmetics. The author's sole purpose is to present consumer information and advice regarding the purchase of makeup. Nowhere herein does the publisher endorse the use of one product over another. The information and recommendations presented strictly reflect the author's opinions, perceptions and knowledge about the subject and products mentioned. Some women may have found success with a particular product that is not recommended or even mentioned herein, or they may be partial to a $250 skin care routine. It is everyone's inalienable right to judge products by their own criteria and standards and to disagree with the author.

More important, because everyone's skin can, and probably will, react to an external stimulus at some time, any product may cause a negative reaction on your skin at one time or another. If you develop a skin sensitivity to a cosmetic, stop using it immediately and consult your physician. If you need medical advice about your skin, it is best to consult a dermatologist.

CHAPTER ONE

Introduction

TALKING ABOUT COSMETICS

It's a jungle out there at the cosmetics counters, and part of the problem is that the language of beauty can be confusing; even simple terms are not always that simple. Therefore, we need to define a few terms before we get into the thick of it. When I use the term "cosmetics," I'm referring to all those skin care and makeup products that are available at the drugstore and cosmetics counters. Skin care products are items that enhance the look or feel of the skin on the face — for example, cleansers, wrinkle creams, moisturizers, masks and astringents. Some skin care products take good care of the face and some of them don't, but I'll get to that later.

Makeup products are items that add color and define the face — for example, lipsticks, eyeshadows and foundations. Again, some of these enhance beauty, and some of them don't. Other buzzwords and expressions will be explained as they come up. My objective at all times is to increase your awareness of the potential obstacles at the cosmetics counters, and to help you avoid these pitfalls whenever possible.

WHAT YOU'LL FIND INSIDE THIS BOOK

Most cosmetics counters have an average of 30 different skin care products and 25 makeup products in dozens of different colors and tones. My books *Blue Eyeshadow Should Be Illegal* and *Blue Eyeshadow Should Still Be Illegal* gave an overview of the cosmetics industry's advertising and promotion techniques. I explained at length why astringents were a waste of money, why wrinkle creams couldn't do what they claimed and why most advertising rhetoric was empty and meaningless. I also described how to tell the difference between blushes, eyeshadows, mascaras and highlighters and how to apply makeup quickly and with fewer products than the salespeople were encouraging you to buy. In essence, almost every page divulged what the cosmetics companies would never reveal to you. The letters of appreciation I've received were all wonderful, encouraging and reinforcing. Most of them sound like this one from a reader in Connecticut:

"First, a hearty thank you for your wonderful book! After having suffered from acne that would not go away and trying just about every antibiotic known to man, not to mention all the cosmetics gimmicks on the market, I feel that I have finally found (thanks to your book) a simple, inexpensive skin care regime. Like you, I was still breaking out in my 30's, trying to dry out my skin with soaps, and suffering from sensitive skin all at the same time! What a difference using the Cetaphil lotion* has made, in addition to the other gentle steps you recommend..."

Nancy J. Fraga

In addition to the compliments, I've received lots of questions about what specific products or cosmetic lines I recommend. It seemed that even after learning how to use a $10 skin care routine that works, how to apply makeup, and what to look for in a particular blush or foundation, women still want to know exactly *which ones* to use. They want to know which foundations go on the lightest, which mascaras don't smudge; which blushes are worth the money, which eyeshadows don't crease, which cosmetics lines are the most reliable and which ones are overpriced. The answers to these questions and more required a radically different kind of research. Although I responded to each letter, truthfully I hadn't yet done the exhaustive (and I mean exhaustive) research necessary to reply to each question thoroughly and accurately. Now I have.

This books presents a product review of the hundreds of cosmetics displayed on department store counters and drugstore racks. Someone had to do it, and, if I was going to live up to my adopted title of the "Ralph Nader of Rouge," I felt it was my responsibility to undertake the task. Not that I was thrilled to do it: I find the cosmetics counters as frustrating, intimidating and annoying as you do. I did not relish the prospect of

---

* The lotion referred to in Nancy Fraga's letter is Cetaphil, a facial cleanser that can be purchased without a prescription at most drugstores. It's great for most skin types and I continue to recommend it over more expensive alternatives.

spending money unnecessarily to test products, nor did I savor the thought of dealing with the salespeople. I knew that most of the information they gave me would be nothing more than sales pitches, hype, anecdotes and scientific cosmebabble. Who wants to put up with that? Not exactly a great way to spend a hundred afternoons. But there was no other way to go about gathering the information for this book.

If you've ever felt uncertain or didn't have the time or energy to figure out for yourself which foundations are too pink or too orange, which eyeshadows are too shiny or too difficult too use, which powders are chalky, which cleansers are too greasy or which toners are too harsh, then product by product and line by line that's what you'll discover in Chapters Six and Seven. Chapter Eight summarizes those reviews, and presents the responses to a survey I mailed to over 500 women about the cosmetics products they use. With this information, you no longer have to rely on your own random search-and-try method or accept the sales clerk's pitch. I have reviewed 25 different major brand-name cosmetics lines and evaluated their products for you. Each product is described in terms of its reliability, value, texture, application and effect.

WHAT ELSE SHOULD BE ILLEGAL BESIDES BLUE EYESHADOW?

Many women who agree with the statement embodied in the title of my first two makeup books want to know what else I think should be "illegal," what else they should avoid besides blue eyeshadow. At the time I wrote those books, there were definitely other items on my "avoid like the plague" list, but if I had added all of them to the title statement, we would have had a very crowded book cover indeed. Following is my complete and updated list of what to avoid. Don't look to the cosmetics industry for confirmation; you won't find it. They want you to buy every one of their products.

All shiny eyeshadows — They make the skin around the eye look wrinkly, even when it's not.

Cream eyeshadows — They tend to go on heavy, crease easily and make blending difficult.

Greasy eye pencils — They are difficult to sharpen, can smudge all over the place, and more often than not, end up looking sloppy and smeared. Not all pencils do this; the thick ones are usually the worst.

All wrinkle creams — These overpriced creams cannot do what they claim and are a pitiful waste of money.

Rejuvenating creams — A wrinkle cream by any other name is still a wrinkle cream.

Astringents — These products irritate the skin. They make oily skin oilier, and they are not capable of closing pores for more than a few minutes, after which the pore returns to its normal shape.

Toners — An astringent by any other name is still an astringent, even if it's low in alcohol or contains "natural" ingredients like lemon or chamomile.

Special eyelid foundations — Most of the time you might as well save your money and use the same foundation and powder you put on your face.

Bright green eyeshadows — Any makeup that is so obvious that you see the makeup and not the woman is always a problem.

Bright blue eye pencils — Less blatant than bright blue eyeshadow, but still too obvious and unattractive.

Eyebrow pencils — I have rarely seen a penciled eyebrow that doesn't look "penciled." And greasy eye pencils are the worst offenders. Do you really want to look like a 1940s woman in the 1990s?

Nonsurgical eyelift creams — If they advertised this one for breasts, would you believe it?

Eyeshadow sets — They waste money, even if you use all the colors (which is rare). Ounce for ounce, the amount of product is smaller than when you buy singly-packaged colors.

Sponge-tip eyeshadow applicators — They tend to wipe off the foundation in the process of applying the eyeshadow; moreover, they drag on the color and make blending difficult. Brushes are almost always better.

Compact-sized brushes — Nobody's eye or cheek is ever that small. Use brushes that are proportional to an adult-size face. This will ease the smooth application of colors.

Models under the age of 30 posing for wrinkle cream ads — This one is self-explanatory.

Models with perfect skin posing for skin care ads in general — This one is also self-explanatory.

Ingredient names no one understands — What good is an ingredient label if we don't understand what it means?

"All day" lipstick claims — After one cup of coffee, you tell me where your lipstick is!

Brown lipsticks — Magazines promote the "nude," "sheer" colors, but what you'll find when you seek them at the cosmetics contours are often brown or brown-orange lipsticks that are anything but nude or sheer. Go for brown lip colors if you want "the dead look."

Brown lipliners — See above.

Mascaras that clump and flake — This one is self-explanatory.

Water-soluble mascaras that don't rinse off completely — Even when they claim to be water-soluble, they're not; you'll see a small black smear under the eye when you're done washing your face.

Eyeshadows that crack — When you near the bottom of the eyeshadow container, the little that is left flakes off and crumbles.

Overly aggressive cosmetics salespeople — Wouldn't it be nice to find a salesperson who doesn't take it as a personal affront when you choose not to buy something?

Poorly lit makeup counters — I sometimes wonder if department stores do this on purpose, so you really can't see yourself clearly.

Miracle ingredients — If you believe this one, I've got a bridge to sell you.

"Dermatologist tested" claims — Unless the test results accompany the claim or you know the dermatologist and the quality of his or her work, this term has no meaning whatsoever. It sounds good, but that's about it.

"Hypoallergenic" claims — No manufacturer can guarantee that you will not breakout or get a rash from using its product.

Hypoallergenic doesn't mean "non-allergenic"; the company just wants you to think so. This is an empty claim that helps sales, not the consumer.

"Non-comedogenic" and "non-acnegenic" claims — Many product labels that make this assertion also list ingredients thought to cause pimples and blackheads. How do companies get away with this one? The Federal Drug Administration (FDA) sets no guidelines for validating such claims. The individual cosmetics companies make that determination. But even if there were guidelines, what may not affect someone else's skin may make your skin break out.

"All natural" claims — I wish I had a nickel for each salesperson who told me certain products were superior because they were all natural and pure. I could list a lot of ingredients that are pure and natural, but that I still wouldn't want to put on my face — or yours! This claim is the most faddish and useless scam around. Consider that the latest genre of products, said to contain "botanicals," but nevertheless includes synthetic ingredients as well. I'm not saying that "natural" means bad, just that it doesn't say anything about the quality or value of the product one way or the other. The same goes for synthetic ingredients. Some are good and some are bad.

Heavy foundations — Foundation that sits on the face like a layer of spackle is unattractive.

Pink- and orange-colored foundations — Foundation that leaves an orange or pink line at the jaw or hairline is unappealing. This is true even when a foundation goes on thin and sheer. Any foundation color that doesn't look like skin tone is a problem.

Tanning powders, bronzers and tinted moisturizers — Although these products give the face a tan appearance, the neck looks pale in comparison. If you try to blend the color down to your neck, it ends up on your collar. Tan, smeared collars are not attractive.

WHY YOU SHOULDN'T GO TO THE COSMETICS COUNTERS ALONE

As you enter the main floor of most department stores, the cosmetics counters are usually the first displays you encounter. The intriguing glass-enclosed showcases sparkle before you. Enticing names and smells suggest elegance and glamour. A plethora of colors radiates from the slick procession of products, beautifully packaged and presented along the counter tops. There are gleaming wet lipsticks, perfectly pressed eyeshadows and glowing blushes arranged in a brilliant array of hues. Each beckons, seeming to guarantee the stunning, vibrant appearance you hope to achieve.

Your hands instinctively reach out to one of the captivating shades of mauve lipstick you have seen on the perfect, pert mouths of the models in the magazines. How velvety and inviting their lips are. They could pout for days; no one could grow tired of looking at their full, generous, luscious mouths. You eagerly search for a tissue to remove the semi-acceptable lipstick you came in with. With a considerate concern about germs and bacteria you discreetly wipe down a sample with the other side of the tissue. The new lipstick glides on with a slick, creamy, sensual feeling. But then you glance in the mirror: before you are blood-red magenta lips.

How did this lipstick color that looked so luscious on the counter turn out so ghastly on your lips? You adjust your head in several directions to see if it's the annoying lighting that is making you look all mouth and no face. Then you begin to tilt the mirror to see if that helps. Then perhaps you dab your tissue to mute the effect. After examining your lips from a dozen different angles you give up and decide to try a different shade or two or three or four. After every failed attempt you wipe off each misjudged lip color until your lips are so swollen, stained and irritated that you can't tell the color from the lips. Finally you give up. There's always the next counter, and plenty of lipsticks at home.

Sound familiar? Another scenario might go something like this: Same department store, same cosmetics counter, same enticing lipsticks, except this time, as you wipe off your lipstick, preparing to apply your newfound dream color, the salesperson approaches. There she is: tall, young, attractive and sporting picture-perfect makeup; she has all the right colors, perfectly blended on disgustingly flawless skin, and a somewhat superior air about her. With a half-interested or over-eager smile she says, "Do you need any help today?"

Exasperated, you reply, "Yes. What do you suggest?"

Quickly, with increased interest and authority, she says, "Oh, that's all wrong for you. Not your color at all. Try this one on — it will be much better for you. But first the lipliner to shape the mouth. Now, that's better already. And it helps immensely if you use a lipstick brush to put your lipstick on. You do have a lipstick brush, don't you?" She deftly applies the lip color she chose and stands back with an appreciative eye. "Now, isn't that better? It's much more your shade. You look beautiful."

"But it's just like the one I came in with."

"But this is moisturizing lipstick. It's designed to protect your lips from the environment. It has a sunscreen, plus vitamin A which will help plump out the lines. It will last all day and keep your lips soft and supple. The pencil will help a lot, too." She stops and grimaces. "You do use a lip pencil, don't you?"

"Do I have to?"

"You can't get lipstick on without it." (Of course how you've been applying lipstick all this time without it is never discussed; it is assumed that up until this point you have been putting lipstick all over your chin and nose.)

Once you are in need of help at the cosmetics counter and someone offers you assistance, from that point on — no matter how you respond — you are most likely to find yourself in trouble. Once you say yes, you might as well turn your pocketbook over at the start, because you'll be introduced to lipliner, gloss and, of course, the latest wrinkle cream. How the subject of wrinkle cream ever comes up will remain forever a mystery, but there it is on the counter, and you find yourself reaching for your wallet. If you decline assistance, you're left to struggle with the choices on your own. You'll no doubt need more tissues, and, come to think of it, maybe the salesperson really does know what colors would look best on you. Damned if you do, and damned if you don't.

This next scenario I call "the nightmare." Same department store, same cosmetics counter, same enticing lipsticks, except this time, as you try to find the right lipstick color, the salesperson who approaches has the worst, most heavily applied makeup you've ever seen — dense foundation with an orange tint, thickly smeared eyeliner and (gasp) the reddest-color blush you've ever seen. You wouldn't want to look like this, even if you were sick. To make matters worse, she's very nice and sounds like she knows what she's talking about. Moreover, she has no intention of letting you test anything on your own; she insists on doing it for you. Then, as soon as she's finished applying your makeup, the other saleswomen emerge from behind the counters and, like a Greek Chorus, gather round and sing the praises of your new look. Of course, as far as you're concerned, you look little better than when you came in, perhaps worse. But what are you going to do — argue the point? If you say you don't like your new look, the women turn to each other in amazement with comments like, "Well, *I* like it," or "*I* think you look great." I can't tell you how many times this production was performed for me while I was researching this book. Every time a salesperson worked on my face, the Chorus chimed in with compliments — sometimes even when, unbeknownst to them, nothing had been applied at all.

Everybody has one of these stories. Regardless of how they are told, the tales all end the same way. Without informed, unbiased advice, it is very tricky to make a wise purchase at a cosmetics counter. When all the information you receive is generated by people with a vested interest in your decision to buy more products, it is practically inevitable that somewhere along the way, you are going to waste money and end up with more than you need. The solution to your every skin care need or makeup problem should not be to buy more.

There are several major obstacles to overcome when tackling the cosmetics buying process: 1) the vast number of choices; 2) the number of products that are nothing more than a waste of time and money; 3) the salespeople who are trained primarily on how to sell products and not how to apply them; and 4) the dilemma of knowing what looks good on you and what doesn't.

Yes, there are a vast number of choices, but this book will help you to narrow down the range relatively faster. Yes, it's hard to know what looks the best and what skin care products work, but it gets easier once you've learned what to avoid. In all honesty, shopping the cosmetics counters may never be an easy experience, but it can be a fun, challenging adventure, and with usable information you can make it just that. This means that you can't go to the cosmetics counters without me — at least not yet.

"Beauty is as beauty buys."

CHAPTER TWO

Behind, In Front of, and Inside the Cosmetics Counters

THE LANGUAGE THAT SELLS MAKEUP

The advertising, marketing and selling techniques used by the cosmetics industry to get consumers to purchase makeup and skin care items are probably the most exaggerated and extreme of any business you'll encounter. When you buy a refrigerator, the chances are fairly good that it will turn on and keep your food cold. If you buy a car, no matter what assertions the salesperson has made about the vehicle, it will probably take you from here to there when you turn it on. (It may break down more then you'd like, but when it works it will take you where you want to go.) The same cannot be said for cosmetics. A moisturizer label that says or implies the product will revitalize, regenerate and rebuild the skin, or prevent wrinkles, or lift and firm cannot fulfill the promise. Astringents and masks that claim to close pores, or give you perfect skin, or perfect anything, will never come through. These products are simply not what they seem, at least not to the extent the manufacturers and salespeople would lead you to believe. That doesn't mean cleaning and moisturizing the skin won't make a positive, wonderful difference to your face — it will. And sunscreens with a Sun Protection Factor (SPF) of 15 or greater will indeed prevent photo-aging when used religiously. But promises of flawless skin made at the cosmetics counters are more fanciful than realistic.

Examining the claims of packaged youth or flawless skin is the most fascinating part of dissecting the cosmetics business. I must point out that there is a stark difference between the things said at the counters and the things said on TV and in magazine ads. Unlike claims made by cosmetics salespeople, which vary wildly from person to person and, as a result, are hard to pin down and refute, cosmetics advertising and promotional literature are bold, unreasonable and in full color. The one- and two-page ads or 30-minute television commercials assert clearly what you are supposed to believe about an individual product or product line. Most of these ads are beautiful and enticing; they have all the trappings of authenticity and veracity. But more often than not, the claims couldn't be further from the truth, or at best they're misleading. What isn't smothered in scientific jargon is shrouded in confusing rhetoric. Anyone who has heard phrases like "a two-week treatment synchronized to your skin's natural rhythm" or "cellular balancing complex" knows that it all sounds good, but no one is quite sure what it means. Are the cells imbalanced? Does skin have a rhythm? And if it does, how does the product play everybody's tune?

In spite of my strong feelings about how women are misled in this area, I feel that to some extent the most flagrant claims of wrinkle-free skin care products have subsided. The FDA in some instances has outlawed deliberate inaccuracies. That doesn't mean advertising departments don't find ways to get around this burden of "truth" by making indirect assertions; furthermore, it is well known that the FDA doesn't have much of a budget to monitor the multibillion dollar cosmetics industry even when companies make blatantly false claims. I'm simply acknowledging that there are some controls out there that are being enforced.

The famous lawsuit that created the latest enforcement guidelines involved endorsements made by the South African heart surgeon Dr. Christian Barnard on behalf of Alfin Fragrances' Glycel skin care line. The FDA contested his claim to inform you "how to grow younger skin," along with similar claims made by Avon, Estee Lauder, Lançome, Christian Dior, Clarins, Orlane, Adrien Arpel, and Germaine Monteil for a handful of their skin care products. To make a long story short, these companies eventually received an ultimatum: Unless they wanted to classify their products as drugs and go through the FDA's scientific procedure to validate their claims, they would have to tone down the language on their labels and ads. The skin care ads now hedge their claims with words such as "appears to," "leaves the skin looking smoother," "changes the appearance of," "lessens the signs of," "reduces the chances of," "reduces the temporary signs of aging." My all-time favorites are such claims as "anti-aging" (as if anyone would buy something that was pro-aging), "affects the visible signs of aging," "reverses the visual damage of aging," "affects the microcirculation of the skin" and "accelerates cell renewal." All moisturizers and exfoliants (scrub products) can make these claims, and there's no law against outrageous pricing and fancy packaging. Just remember that nothing specific, long-lasting or permanent can be guaranteed because nothing specific, long-lasting or permanent can be proved.

Many cosmetics companies produce elaborate four-color brochures touting the special effects of their skin care products. These "scientifically-generated" promotions are often accompanied by very official-looking test charts and diagrams. The layouts are most impressive in their technical dramatization and clinical appearance; they are produced by graphic artists and marketing departments rather than by bona fide scientists in a neutral laboratory. They amount to little more then pretty pictures with enigmatic headings and descriptions. Even when illustrations do represent a scientific study of some type, there are still important questions to ask regarding the test results. Take, for example, a brochure that depicts a microscopic section of skin before and after a product was applied. The manufacturer is trying to demonstrate that when water is retained in the skin over a period of time, the skin is measurably more elastic. But a microscopic picture of skin that shows improvement after a cream is applied, or a graph depicting a similar change, in and of itself is meaningless.

You are given no information about the condition of the skin before the cream was applied, how old the test subject or subjects were, how many people (or animals) were tested, and whether the results were uniform among all the subjects. You don't know who performed the test, whether double-blind scientific procedures were used, who analyzed the results, how long the effects lasted, and if the results were the same for a placebo cream placed on another part of the skin. There is no way those pictures or graphs have any legitimate scientific significance whatsoever.

It is illegal for a cosmetics company to claim that its cosmetics (with the exception of those containing a sunscreen) can change, alter or effect permanent structural change in the status of the skin — because they don't. Cosmetics don't change the skin permanently; that's why they're called *cosmetics*. If you listen carefully, you'll see that most manufacturers don't state directly that their products cause permanent alterations — they imply it. They say their products "revitalize," "repair," "firm," "plump," "nourish," "re-energize" and "restore." They call the products "skin regulators," "night repair," "skin recovery creams," "equalizers" and "skin defenders." These words are all permissible, provided the product contains ingredients such as oil or propylene glycol that can keep water in the skin — something all moisturizers do to one extent or another. Whenever I see these terms, I'm reminded of something provocative I once heard a dermatologist say: "To think that a moisturizer with herbs, vitamins, botanicals or some other skin care ingredient can feed the skin, would be like thinking that you can rub blood on your face and get a transfusion." Not a pretty picture, but it makes the point nicely.

Cosmetics companies are permitted to use words that make it sound as if their products can perform medical miracles and heal the skin: "cell extracts," "serum" (sounds like a blood transfusion), "placental extracts," "hyaluronic acid," "retinol" (sounds like Retin-A, doesn't it?), "living water serum," "collagen" and "elastin." Of course, there is no proof that any of these ingredients can do anything but soften the skin or help it retain water.

The words that sound scientific are often the most presumptuous and carry the least information. I've yet to find a salesperson who, when pressed, can define "micro-refining," "micro-targeted," "micro-bubbles," "isotonic energy," "bio-synergetic," "bio-performance" and "micro-lipid-concentrate." Often these terms have been created by the company to sound impressive, but that's about as far as it goes.

Then there are the untranslatable foreign words: "multi-Regenerante," "hydro-serum" (sounds like a hydro-blood transfusion this time), "lipo-serum," "multi-reparateur restructurant," "resultante Creme," "hydra-systeme" (water system?), "synchro serum" and "hydrafilm." Who knows for sure what they mean?

The technical terms designed to create the image of protecting the skin from environmental threats — "skin defender," for example, and the claims "eliminates free radical damage" or "eliminates environmental damage" — usually apply to products that contain a sunscreen or an antioxidant. Inclusion of these ingredients allows companies to claim that the product in question protects the skin from the elements. Unfortunately, unless the sunscreen is rated 15 or higher, it cannot protect the skin adequately from the damaging rays of the sun, and most of these products contain an SPF of only 4 to 8. If antioxidants are included in the products, these ingredients remain on the surface of the skin and merely keep the air off the face.

The terminology applied to products that supposedly ward off acne is less varied, but the general ad approach is the same. It attempts to convince the consumer that certain formulations can correct oily or combination skin because they are any and all of the following: "dermatologist tested," "allergy tested," "laboratory tested," "non-comedogenic," "oil-free," "natural," and "designed for sensitive skins." All of that sounds great, but the words can't guarantee that your skin won't react adversely to the product or that the product will keep you from developing acne or even change the acne you do have. I've stated before that although there are no absolutes about what elements cause acne or blackheads, there are ingredients that are considered to be a higher risk than others. As surprising as this sounds, despite what the label says, some "non-comedogenic" products contain components that may exacerbate blackheads and acne.

All of these advertising terms make an appeal to our emotions — those of us who want to believe that we can win the battle against the clock or against acne. Even if the product provides only a temporary victory, most people feel that it is better than no victory at all. This sliver of hope, and the sensational allure of skin care ads, keep many people, especially women, hooked on spending a lot of money on skin care and makeup products in general. The satisfaction they obtain is emotional rather than physical.

Imagine two women with the same genetic background and health status; both have normal skin and they tan on a regular basis without a sunscreen. One of the women uses skin care products from the drugstore. The other uses every product Chanel makes for her skin type. Both women will develop wrinkles at nearly the same rate. Now imagine the same two women: one uses drugstore products and the other uses Chanel as before, but in this case the one who uses the drugstore products never tans and is diligent about wearing a sunscreen with an SPF of 15 or greater, and the one who uses Chanel tans on a regular basis without the use of a potent sunscreen. The woman using the drug store products will have almost wrinkle-free skin, whereas her counterpart with the $500 skin care routine will have a substantial amount of wrinkles by the age of 40.

The major problem with this advertising and marketing verbiage is that we want to believe it all. What woman over the age of 35 doesn't want to have her skin firmed and restructured? Who doesn't want to believe that there are scientists in the Swiss Alps or in some fancy laboratory designing products that can rid us of wrinkles? After all, if I can fax a letter to Australia in less than a minute, and satellites can bring me live, up-to-the-minute coverage of world events, surely the technology exists to make skin look younger. Sigh. If I thought for one second that there was a moisturizer or astringent or specialty cream that could truly change the wrinkles on my skin or close a pore, I'd buy it for myself, recommend it to you, and buy stock in the company that makes it. To a large extent, it is our *willingness to believe* that drives the marketing hype behind each of these products. It is only our commitment to reality and a raised consumer awareness that will prevent us from buying products that can't possibly do what they say. The first step is to stop being deluded by slick packaging and advertisements.

INGREDIENTS YOU NEED AND DON'T NEED FOR DRY SKIN

Although there are many products that don't make any sense, there are many products that are quite beneficial, and even important, for the skin. After defusing the claims, promises and company effusion, most of us know that skin care is important, which is a major reason why we keep buying cleansing and moisturizing products. In Chapter Seven, I'll review specific products from each line. In this section I'll briefly list the most beneficial ingredients to look for in skin care products. None of these ingredients is a miracle, and none prevents skin from aging — except for sunscreens — or cures acne and blackheading. Keeping water in the skin is the key to "younger-appearing" skin, because dehydrated skin looks older. Gently exfoliating the skin and using a mild disinfectant will help control acne and blackheading. It can be just that simple, regardless of how complicated the cosmetic companies try to make it sound.

It is important to note that all the ingredients listed below exist naturally, are synthetically produced or are extracted from animal or plant tissue. Regardless of the components or how a product is manufactured (even substances found in human skin), no cosmetic cream can become a permanent part of your skin. Whether synthetic or natural ingredients are better for your skin is irrelevant, since all products include both. There are very few, if any, 100 percent natural skin care products on the market. Besides, there is no way to tell from the ingredient label alone which ingredients are natural and which ones are synthetic.

The most beneficial ingredients in products designed for dry skin to look for are:

> Allantoin, Amino Acids, Proteins (Hydrolyzed Animal Protein), Caprylic/Capric/Lauric Triglycerides, Cholesterol, Phospho-lipids (Lecithin), Collagen, Elastin, Fatty Acids (Stearic Acid),

Hyaluronic Acid, Lanolin, Liposomes, Mucopolysaccharides, Glycosaminoglycans, Oil (petrolatum, mineral oil, jojoba oil, squalane, lanolin oil, avocado oil, egg oil, palm oil, sunflower seed oil, sweet almond oil, carrot oil, sandalwood oil, rice bran oil, macadamia oil, coconut oil, basil oil, castor oil (yes even castor oil), Propylene Glycol, Butylene Glycol, Polyethylene Glycol (PEG), Glycerin, Sodium PCA, Tocopherol and water.

The ingredients I've listed above can help maintain soft, moist skin. There is no guarantee, however, that you won't be allergic to one or many of them. There is also no guarantee that any or all of them will make a difference on your skin. The likelihood is that if your moisturizer contains one or more of these, and most of them do, it can make a difference. If your skin is dry, your skin can feel softer and look smoother for as long as you use the product. But the effect lasts only as long as you use the product. Once it is washed off or absorbed into the skin, the effect is gone. If your skin is not dry there is little to no benefit gained from using a moisturizer that contains any of these ingredients.

The above ingredients are found in moisturizers in all price ranges. I recommend that you experiment with lower-priced products before venturing into the range above $15. If the less expensive ones can work just as well — and they do — why bother with the high-end stuff? If your skin looks good, what difference does it make how little you spend on skin care or makeup?

By the way, there are a large range of ingredients with very technical-sounding names that are used to create and maintain an attractive, pleasant, creamy consistency in moisturizers and other cosmetics. Cetyl alcohol, ceteareth, cetearyl alcohol, polysorbates, myristyl alcohol and stearyl alcohol, are just a few of them. Unless you're allergic to them, they won't do you any harm. They're basic components of almost every cosmetic you buy.

Some ingredients that get quite a bit of dramatic attention, and increase the price of a product considerably, have no ability to help your skin retain moisture and thus don't make you look a minute younger; these are, at best, useless. They aren't harmful in any way; they just aren't helpful.

The ingredients to avoid or disregard in products designed for dry skin are:

Adenosine Triphosphate, Algae Extract, Amniotic Fluid, Animal Thymus Extract, Animal Tissue Extract, Neural Lipid Extract,

Epidermal Lipid Extract, Serum Albumin, Serum Protein, Spleen Extract, Tissue Matrix Extract, Vitamin A*, Retinyl Palmitate*, and Retinol*.

INGREDIENTS YOU NEED AND DON'T NEED FOR OILY SKIN

There is much controversy and disagreement over what works on oily, acne-prone skin. Those who have this skin condition already have experienced the endless search for products that will improve the skin. Although ads lead you to believe that specially designed products for oily skin zap zits or dry up oil, the truth is that many of them can't do either reliably. Anyone who has ever used them knows this.

The ingredients listed below are considered to be soothing, cleansing or antiseptic for oily skin. They are also, for the most part, considered ingredients that won't cause blackheads. They may or may not work on your skin; there's no way to know in advance because an individual's skin reacts differently to the same ingredients.

The most beneficial ingredients in products designed for oily skin to look for are:

Allantoin, Ammonium Glycerhizinate, Butylene Glycol, Propylene Glycol, Polyethylene Glycol, Hexylene Glycol, Glycerin, Kaolin, Bentonite, Sodium Laureth Sulfate and Magnesium Laureth Sulfate.

It is harder to heal an oily, acned skin condition than we would like to believe, but that's the painful truth. There are steps you can take to calm down acne as well as steps you shouldn't take. But you can't completely eliminate the problem with products from the cosmetics counters or the drugstore — those of us who have acne have come to understand this.

Naming ingredients to avoid if you have oily skin is fairly controversial. Some of you are using products right now that contain several of these ingredients, and you may feel that your skin is doing just fine. So much

---

*These ingredients are are derivatives of Vitamin A, as is the prescription drug Retinoic Acid (better known as Retin-A). This association with Retin-A misleads many consumers into believing that products containing Vitamin A, retinyl palmitate and retinol provide the same or similar benefits to the skin as Retin-A. None of the claims are proven. Retin-A is a prescription drug, and its effects — both positive and negative — are quite potent. You would not want a cosmetic to have the same effects.

for tests, and so much for my opinion. As I said, this is a complicated, tricky area of skin care. But if your skin is not doing well or you are experiencing skin irritation and you're wondering what to do about it, you may want to start by eliminating some products that contain the questionable ingredients in this list.

I can personally attest that skin care products containing irritating ingredients are usually more harmful than helpful. So the list below contains ingredients that are recognized by most dermatologists and cosmetics chemists to cause breakouts — such as lanolin and isopropyl myristate — and those ingredients that I feel make oily skin worse — such as alcohol and camphor — because of the irritation they can cause.The ingredients to avoid or disregard in products designed for oily skin if you are experiencing skin irritation:

> Acetone, Benzalkonium Chloride, Benzoyl Peroxide, Camphor, Isopropyl Myristate, Lanolin, Lanolin Alcohol, Lanolin Acid, Isopropyl Lanolate, Acetylated Lanolin, Salicylic Acid, SD Alcohol, Sodium Lauryl Sulfate (if it is among the first ingredients listed), Zinc Lauryl Sulfate, Ammonium Lauryl Sulfate, Magnesium Lauryl Sulfate and Witch Hazel.

INGREDIENTS YOU NEED AND DON'T
NEED FOR SENSITIVE SKIN

First of all, let me state plainly that to one extent or another we all have sensitive skin. Do not skip over this section because you think you have a tough exterior. At some time almost all of us will experience a skin reaction to something. You can prevent some skin reactions, however, if you are aware of what often causes them.

The best part of the cosmetics world is that many of the products just feel so good on the skin. The silky smooth texture of creams and lotions gliding over the skin and leaving a dewy moist gloss behind can make the skin look and feel beautiful and provide a blissful emotional lift as well. Same thing with makeup; as you artfully, or even not so artfully, apply an appealing shade of eyeshadow to your lid in a velvety soft tone that sets off the depth of your eyes perfectly, you may feel a surge of self-esteem as you admire the way you look. Now that's what makeup should be all about. Unfortunately, for those of you with even slightly sensitive skin, finding products that enhance and don't irritate is indeed a challenge. I would love to list ingredients that I could guarantee won't cause your skin to flare up, but there is no single ingredient or combination of ingredients that can live up to that sweeping claim. Numerous combinations exist, in all sorts of combinations, but what they can do to your skin — their claims to be "hypoallergenic" or "dermatologist tested" notwithstanding — is anyone's guess. Your only recourse, and this is not the best news, is to keep experimenting until you find what works for you. Consult your dermatologist if you do get a reaction, return the products that are suspect, and keep track of the ingredients included in products to which you seem to be allergic.

For example, many preservatives present in almost all cosmetics are not good for skin and are known to cause allergic reactions. But chemists have few options when it comes to preventing microbes from taking up residence in their products. Fragrances are another known source of skin irritations, and often they are used simply to mask the unpleasant odor of many cosmetics ingredients. But more often than not, particularly in cosmetics that have strong, noticeable scents, fragrances are used to increase sales. It appears that many cosmetics consumers want their lotions and creams to exude an obvious bouquet. That isn't the fault of the cosmetics companies, although it does reflect a need for consumer education. If you want perfume, use perfume. But choose skin care products that are fragrance-free!

Then there are the ingredients that are helpful but are still potential skin irritants — sunscreens, lanolin and urea. Individual ingredients like these may possibly react alone or in concert with other ingredients on every type of skin and under every type of condition. It would be impossible to predict with any accuracy what, where, when and how a single ingredient in one of any number of products will affect your skin. When you consider the hundreds of chemicals a woman places on her face in such varied products as cleansers, toners, moisturizers, foundations, blushes, lipsticks, eyeshadows and mascaras, it is surprising to realize how really safe and non-irritating cosmetics usually are.

I'm sure that many of you already are aware of this, but it can never be said too often: If you have an allergic reaction of any kind to a cosmetic product, stop using it immediately and consult your physician if the problem persists. Do not hesitate to return the product to the place where you purchased it and get your money back. It is not your fault that the product caused you problems. Also, returning the product gives the cosmetics company essential information about how their formulas are working.

THE CRAZY THINGS SALESPEOPLE SAY

Salespeople in general say the most amazing, contrived things, and why should those in the cosmetics industry be any different? As I made my way across this country shopping for cosmetics (I traveled to nine major cities to research this book), the conversations I had with cosmetics salespeople were, more often than not, frustrating and ridiculous. Many of the things they said — with such earnest conviction — had no basis in fact or reality. In all fairness, I should say that there were times when the salespeople were honest, straightforward, even-tempered, caring, helpful and, on occasion, talented makeup artists. Some actually made some suggestions that were helpful or recommended inexpensive products or products in other lines that they thought would be what I was looking for. Several of the salespeople I interviewed admitted that they didn't understand the sales rhetoric they were trained to repeat. A few salespeople talked candidly about the products they were selling. I cannot express to you how much I appreciated such openness and honesty. They were a breath of hype-free air. Unfortunately, such conversations were the exceptions, not the rule. I encountered indifference or rudeness when it became clear that I wasn't willing to buy right then and there. I found extreme sales pressure almost everywhere I went. Salespeople brooded if I didn't like the makeup application I received and were irritated if I questioned "facts." It is not surprising that the cosmetics section at most department stores is referred to, unaffectionately, as "Barracuda Bay."

I should mention now that well trained salespeople are not necessarily assets to consumers, but they are not always detrimental, either. On the up side, sales staff who are not well trained can't overtalk products they know nothing about. On the down side, people who are not well trained are less able to help you with color and product choices. Well trained salespeople can provide a great service, so long as you are able to ignore their infuriating sales-training expressions.

Here are some typical conversations I had while shopping for makeup over the past year:

CONVERSATION 1

Saleswoman: *This foundation will last you at least a year.*

Me: *How is that possible when the last time I bought it, it only lasted five months?*

Saleswoman: *You were probably using it incorrectly. You only need the tiniest amount.*
Me: *Do you think I have too much foundation on now?*
Saleswoman: *Well, no.*
Me: *If I cut back any more, I won't have any on at all!*

CONVERSATION 2

Saleswoman: *These products are developed and formulated in Switzerland. Everyone knows the Swiss and the Europeans know more about skin care than we do. They take much better care of their skin than we do.*
Me: *Have you ever been to Europe?*
Saleswoman: *No.*
Me: *Funny, when I was in France the women behind the cosmetics counters there said the same thing about American products and American women. Did you know that almost all of the major American cosmetic lines sold here are sold there? Do you think it's possible that they take such good care of their skin because of American products instead of the other way around?*
Saleswoman: *I don't think that's possible.*
Me: *What don't you think is possible, that they sell American products in Europe or that European women buy American products?*

CONVERSATION 3

Saleswoman: *All of our lipsticks are hand flamed to give them this beautiful long-lasting sheen.*
Me: *Most lipsticks are hand flamed or mechanically flamed to create that finished look, but that has no effect on the way the product will last. It is strictly aesthetic.*
Saleswoman: *The quilting finish on our eyeshadows will prevent chipping and flaking.*
Me: *But your demo here is flaking and chipping. How do you explain that?*
Saleswoman: *Well, it's just a demo; it's not the real thing.*
Me: *It sure looks real to me.*
Saleswoman: *Our products are all made in a dust-free environment.*
Me: *Dust free? Does dust affect the quality of a product? And how do you suppose they control dust, given the nature of powders and talcs?*
Saleswoman: *They just do!*

CONVERSATION 4

Saleswoman: *Not one of our eyeshadows is shiny.*

Me: *Most of these colors look very shiny to me.*

Saleswoman: *They look shiny, but they're not really. They go on totally matte.*

Me (after trying one or two shades on the back of my hand): *This still looks pretty shiny to me.*

Saleswoman: *That's not shine; it's just silky looking. You know, luminescent. It goes on silky, not shiny.*

Me (staring in astonishment): *You're telling me this looks matte to you? Excuse me — "luminescent" and not shiny? You really sell these as non-iridescent to people who are looking for matte shadows?*

Saleswoman: *If that's what they want.*

(I imagine that when a customer requests shiny shadows that these same colors automatically become shiny not luminescent.)

CONVERSATION 5

Saleswoman: *All of our products contain botanicals. They are totally natural. Botanicals have been used for thousands of years. Even the Egyptians used them.*

Me: *But the Egyptians didn't live long. Life expectancy back then was maybe 30 years and Cleopatra died at 16. That doesn't say much for botanicals, now does it?*

CONVERSATION 6

Saleswoman: *We're not legally allowed to say what this product really can do, because of FDA regulations. We can only say that it will smooth the skin and make it softer, but it does much more. Our studies prove that this cream can get rid of almost all those fine lines around your eyes and keep them from coming back. But, legally I can't say that.*

Me: *Why do you think the FDA wants to prevent you from revealing the truth about your wrinkle cream?*

Saleswoman: *It has to do with how cosmetics are legally classified. Cosmetics require different regulations than prescription items.*

Me: *Cosmetics require less testing than prescription drugs and the cosmetics companies don't won't to spend the time or money putting their products under the scrutiny of the FDA. Because if they did, and the product didn't do what it said it could do, that would be a lot of money wasted. And given that the cosmetics companies tend to come up with "new, improved" formulas every year, they would have wasted millions on products that didn't stay on the market very long.*

CONVERSATION 7

Saleswoman: *You should always wear a moisturizer under your makeup to protect your face from the foundation.*

Me: *Why does my face need to be protected from your foundation? Is there something wrong with your foundation?*

Saleswoman: *No, it's just that the foundation contains coloring agents that are best kept away from the skin.*

Me: *But I thought foundations are designed to stay on top of the skin and not absorb into the skin?*

CONVERSATION 8

Saleswoman: *Skin ages the most at night, which is why you need a very good night cream for the delicate skin around your eyes.*

Me: *But I thought that skin ages mostly during the day, as a result of sun exposure. Isn't that why sunscreens are touted for preventing the skin from aging, while no other cosmetics are allowed to make the same claim?*

Saleswoman: *(No response)*

THE NEW COSMETICS COUNTER —
TELEVISION COSMETICS TALK SHOWS

Ever since I got cable television I've enjoyed flipping through the channels to see what's on all forty stations. Sometimes this hypnotizes me, and I begin using the remote control compulsively and mindlessly. Once in a while, an info-commercial snaps me out of this state, but I'm not thankful. The consumer reporter in me always becomes incensed. You are all probably familiar with those half-hour television commercials that look like talk shows and sound like talk shows but are nothing more than paid advertisements for everything from spot removers and kitchen accessories to get-rich-quick deals. Given the variety and sheer repetition of these "programs" (and I use that word loosely), I must assume that a large number of people call the flashing toll-free numbers to spend their hard-earned money. And that outrages me, because I know that these shows are so completely misleading, one-sided and biased that it would be impossible for a consumer to make an intelligent decision based on the information presented.

The info-commercials that upset me the most are those that sell makeup and skin care products — particularly a certain product line of creams, lotions and some kind of enzyme supplement that is supposed to eliminate cellulite. It is impossible to remove cellulite with a pill or cream of any kind; furthermore, the FDA has informed me that they are working to prohibit the airing of these ads. The specific info-commercial to which I refer (although they all do this) features endorsements from women who claim to have used the advertised products with miraculous results. The show features a "doctor" (a Ph.D. maybe?) in a lab coat who recommends the products wholeheartedly. In my many years research- ing the cosmetics industry, I have yet to find an independent doctor who will suggest that there is any possible way to get rid of cellulite with creams or vitamins. I can't think of a bigger waste of time and money than beating or massaging your thighs with a cream or lotion in order to get rid of cellulite.

Another television cosmetics line is brought to you by the Victoria Jackson Company. The salespeople "behind the counter" of this info- commercial are an attractive pair of actresses, a very assertive Elizabeth Baxter-Birney, and a rather passive, albeit smiling, Ali McGraw. Both of these women, who are paid for their time and endorsements, claim to be Victoria Jackson converts. As a result of discovering her products, they have been able to toss away all of their other cosmetics. During the "show," Elizabeth and Ali interview Victoria Jackson about her remark- able products, which she describes repeatedly as totally "sheer, light and natural." This commercial, although somewhat less irritating than the one for cellulite, is a very slick advertising vehicle and, if the number of buyers is as high as the program claims, the line is doing very well. But shopping for makeup via television is not a good idea. Without being able to test the products, read the ingredient label, or see the product for yourself, you will not get a bargain, especially not at $120 a pop. I review the specific products from the Victoria Jackson line in Chapter Six.

All of these paid-for "talk" shows that look like legitimate programming are nothing more than long advertisements. They are not objective; the people in the audiences do not give unsolicited endorsements. The shows are ads, designed to create an image of truth and validity, and they do not provide you with the viewpoints of consumer advocates, as would any real program. My opinion? Save your money. Television is not the place to buy makeup or skin care products. I know it's inviting to pick up a phone and take care of your desire to feel beautiful, but be strong and switch to another channel.

Conversation overheard between two cosmetics saleswomen:

"I wonder if any of this stuff works?"
"Of course it's working; it's paying my rent."

CHAPTER THREE

An Eye On Beauty: Shopping for Cosmetics

GETTING THROUGH THE JUNGLE

The only way to survive the 1990s at the cosmetics counters is to change the way you've shopped for cosmetics in the past. What I'm about to tell you is going to sound familiar, and some of it is going to sound like a pain in the you-know-what, but if you follow my advice you'll be you much less likely to leave the store with something you don't want, don't like or can't afford. Even if you take to heart only one of the following lessons, you are likely to be a happier cosmetics consumer.

✓ First you must be willing to change some of your beliefs about the world of skin care and makeup. A cosmetics company does not necessarily have your best interest at heart. As is true with most businesses, a cosmetic company's interest is the bottom line, and what you buy affects that bottom line. If you are willing to buy stuff that is overpriced, doesn't work or isn't fashionable, they will keep selling it, because there is no reason for them to change. No one's pores have ever been closed by using a toner, and no wrinkle has gone away by using a wrinkle cream, but we continue to buy toners and wrinkle creams. So why should the cosmetics companies stop selling them?

✓ The question I am asked most often is: "What cosmetics line do you like the most?" I truly wish it were that simple. If I could put my energy into one or two lines that I thought were good enough to recommend to everyone, believe me I would. Regrettably, that is not the case. Every cosmetics line has good and bad products, some more bad than others. For the sake of emphasis, I will repeat: Every cosmetics line has good and bad products. That includes skin care items as well as makeup. I have yet to find a cosmetics line anywhere in the world that is 100 percent or even 60 percent wonderful. All lines have their share of useless, overly perfumed, glaringly shiny and unreliable products. They also have products that work, but I will get to those specifics in chapters Six and Seven.

✓ Do not assume that one line is automatically better than another, particularly when many of the companies are owned by the same parent company. What is probably closer to the truth is that there are a few products in every line that might work for you. It is great when you find a line that you are comfortable with. For example, you might like Prescriptives lipsticks or love Clinique foundations. But that does not mean that every other product in those lines are also guaranteed to please you or be good for you. No matter how enthusiastic salespeople are about their terrific line, remember that they could very well have been saying the same thing about a different line last week.

✓ You do not and should not buy impulsively or quickly. You can take notes, wear a color for a while, take a sample of a skin care item, and then make a decision. In fact, buying a product you've just tried on and haven't worn for at least an hour or two, is almost always a mistake. You have nothing to lose if you take your time and consider your purchase. How does it look in different light? How does it look and feel after it's been on your face for a while? I cannot tell you how many women I watched buying foundations after looking at them in store light that was little better than a dimly lit restaurant.

✓ Cosmetics advertising may be alluring and interesting, but they are ads, not documentaries. Just because the ads are sensual, that doesn't mean the products featured in the ads are sensual, and it doesn't mean they'll make you more sensual. Accept seductive ads for what they are — seductive ads.

✓ Cosmetics advertising is very powerful and can strongly affect the way we make decisions at the cosmetics counters. I know that sounds simple-minded, but it would also be foolish to ignore the fact that advertising sells products. Oil of Olay is my favorite example. There isn't a plant or animal or place called "Olay"; there are no ingredients called "Olay"; yet Oil of Olay has had a tremendously impressive sales record, and most people know the product by name. Next time you think you are not affected by cosmetics advertising, think again.

✓ Figure out your cosmetics budget and stick to it. There are excellent products available in all price ranges. Salespeople can be both helpful and intimidating at the same time. It is their job to find products that are supposed to help you with whatever skin problem you have or that you want to prevent. A good cosmetics salesperson can sell you a line of skin care products for $200 before you know it. You'd like to think you're stronger than that and aren't capable of overspending to that extent, but we've all done it, and many of us have done it more than once. Admitting that you are one of the weak ones in this regard, and setting some solid, non-negotiable limits on what you are willing to buy, is your first step. The second step is sticking to it.

✓ Consider the basic cost of what you are buying. When you break down the cost of a product and evaluate it in dollars per pound as opposed to dollars per ounce, you will start seeing the absurdity of cosmetics pricing. The cost of beauty: La Prairie's Creme Cellulair is about $1,900 a pound; Stendahl's Emulsion Base Moisturizer costs $400 a pound; Christian Dior's Base Fluid costs $250 a pound and Neutragena's Moisture costs $40 per pound. Now you tell me, which one do you choose, given that you know they all can do practically the same thing for the skin and contain similar ingredients?

✓ I know I've said this before, but more than anything else it bears repeating: There are no miracle ingredients, patented products, trade secrets, exotic ingredients or doctor-tested formulas that will permanently change the appearance of wrinkles or keep the skin from wrinkling (this does not apply to sunscreens or Retin-A). If there were a magic potion, it wouldn't stay under wraps. Chemists are capable of analyzing a product's ingredients, duplicating whatever they want. Sophisticated technologies make reproduction of a product's components as easy as assembling a jigsaw puzzle when all the pieces are included. If there were one wrinkle cream that worked, it wouldn't take long for a million copies to show up on the market right behind it. (The reason there is only one Retin-A is because Johnson & Johnson owns the exclusive patent on it and not because it is a secret. Everyone knows what's in Retin-A and what makes it work. When the duration of that patent has expired there will be dozens of generic Retin-As on the market in a flash.)

✓ Mascaras, foundations, lipsticks, blushes and eyeshadows from expensive lines have the same basic ingredients as those in the less expensive lines. Let me say that again for emphasis: Most cosmetic products, regardless of price or packaging, have more in common than they have differences. Formulations might vary and there are those products that are better than others, but on the whole, I found just as many great products at the drugstore as I did at the department store. Marketing creates the mystique of makeup. If spending $50 on foundation makes you look $50 better, then I guess it's worth it. But if spending $50 makes you look the same as if you had spent $10, then I would recommend you reconsider your decision process.

SHOPPING FOR COSMETICS IN A DEPARTMENT STORE

There is something very intimidating yet elegant about shopping for cosmetics in a department store. The sales pressure is evident from the moment you approach the glass-and-chrome cases outlining the cosmetics area. The elegance lies in the pampered feeling you get from the earnest, helpful information and advice the salespeople provide. How can you have your cake and eat it too? How can you enjoy the luxury of the service without taking a bath in purchases? The following directives are essential to surviving makeup shopping:

✓ Know ahead of time what you need or want. If you're looking for a lipstick, you should not leave with a mascara, eye cream and lip liner.

✓ Have a mirror with you so that you can leave the store — yes, I said leave the store — and look at yourself in the daylight. Never trust the interior lighting in the store. At almost every cosmetics counter the lighting is like a bad joke. No matter how you stretch your face toward the light or adjust the mirror, it just isn't going to reflect what you need to see.

✓ If you are trying to match colors to a particular outfit, bring part of the outfit with you. Yes, it's a pain to schlep it, but the benefits of getting the right color outweigh the inconvenience.

✓ If the salesperson or the brochures accompanying a product make claims about what you should expect after using the product, ask if you can return the product if it doesn't do whatever it is supposed to do. It is the best way to guarantee your satisfaction. Do not hesitate to return a product that doesn't live up to its claim — regardless of what the claim is. If the "signs of aging" don't go away, if the all-day lipstick barely makes it through the first coffee-break, if the creaseless eyeshadow creases and the shine-proof foundation shines, if the toner doesn't "refine" your pores and the promise of flawless skin is flawed, take it all back for a refund!

✓ Remember that the salesperson does not necessarily know anything about makeup artistry or skin care. While researching cosmetics counters, I encountered many salespeople who chose the wrong foundation for me or selected skin care products that were inappropriate for my skin type. Quite often different products from the same cosmetic line would be recommended by different salespeople. What happens at the cosmetics counters often has nothing to do with expertise and everything to do with ringing up sales.

✓ If you are shopping for a foundation, do not wear a foundation to the store, or be prepared to take it off. Never, absolutely never, test a makeup product over the makeup you are wearing. If you can't persuade yourself to enter a store without wearing makeup, then use the moisturizer demos that are displayed on the counter to help rub it off when you get there.

✓ Testing cosmetics is, in my opinion, one of the most important ways to discover what works best for you and what doesn't. But this is indeed a controversial issue. Concern over bacteria and germs is valid. There are a few companies that offer small, individually-packaged demo brushes; these neat giveaways, however, are not always available, and so you can't count on being able to use them. There are cotton balls and cotton swabs available at most counters, but unfortunately, they are terrible applicators for makeup. Taking your own brushes is an option, but that makes things problematic for the next customer. Regardless of what you choose to do, always ask for clean demo brushes first. If they are not available, then use a cotton ball, cotton swab or your fingers to apply the makeup so that you can at least estimate how the product will look on you. Once home, use a sponge to apply foundation and full-sized brushes to apply eyeshadows and blushes.

✓ Do not test colors on the back of your hand except when you're comparing colors to narrow down your choices. After selecting the colors that seem to blend well with your skin, or that look like what you had in mind, take the time to apply them on your face.

✓ Always ask if you can have a sample of the product to try at home. More and more frequently, there are free samples available at cosmetics counters.

SHOPPING FOR COSMETICS IN A DRUGSTORE

When I started reviewing drugstore cosmetics lines, I was surprised how much I liked the experience of shopping for cosmetics without anyone attempting to sell me products I didn't need or want. That was particularly true for skin care products. The frustration occurred when I was shopping for makeup items. Because of the way drugstore makeup products are displayed and packaged, the colors and textures are difficult to see, so there is no way to know exactly what you're buying.

Many drugstore products I tried were excellent, but there are rarely testers available, much less free samples, so most of the time you are stuck guessing how a makeup color will look on you. Occasionally, I have seen cosmetics tester units at the drugstore, but they're not used consistently from store to store. Most of the product colors are displayed through clear plastic; seeing the color is helpful, but how it will look on your skin is uncertain. There are also products — lip pencils and eye pencils for example — where you can't see the color at all. In these cases, names or color swatches — and we all know how reliable they are — are the only references you can go by. Even simple names like "brown" or "pink" have a wide range of variations.

My suggestions in the product review section will help, but to know how a product will really look on you, you'll have to wait until you get home. When you consider the expensive department store alternatives, it's often worth the risk. A bag of cosmetics costing $60 at the drugstore could contain 15 or 20 products, while at the department store $60 worth of cosmetics might only include three to five. The pros and cons are obvious, but what should you do? My basic suggestion is that there are some products that it makes no sense to buy at the department store, and others it makes no sense to buy at the drugstore.

The most difficult item to buy at the drugstore is foundation. I almost never recommend buying foundation that you can't try on and check in the daylight, but again there are some suggestions in Chapter Six that will help if the cosmetics counters are just too expensive for your budget. Lipsticks and eyeshadows can be tricky items to buy at the drugstore. Although I found that many cosmetics lines at the drugstore had excellent lipstick choices, it is very hard to judge how the color will end up looking on your lips. For those women who already have a good sense of what colors look best on them, the drugstore is a great place to shop for lipstick; for those who aren't sure, go back to the department store. The problem with buying eyeshadows at the drugstore is the paltry selection of matte colors; most are just too shiny to recommend. But if you choose to wear shiny eye colors, (although by now I hope I've talked you out of that fashion no-no), there is absolutely no reason to pay $15 for them at the department store when you can buy the same thing for $3 at the drugstore.

There is never a reason to buy mascara at the department store — the prices are absurd. I found several wonderful mascaras at the drugstore that were as good as, if not superior to, many of the department store brands I tested. This is also true for lip pencils and some eye pencils. The colors of lip pencils are fairly standard, as are the texture and wearability. Eye pencils are more problematic, but some of the ones at the drugstore are identical to the ones at the department store. There is no reason to spend more than $3 to $5 on a pencil; any more is a blatant waste of money. If you follow my advice in the makeup review section you will discover this for yourself.

Concealers are also something you can buy at the drugstore. Many of the concealers I saw at the department store cosmetics counters were too dark, too peach, pink or rose. The consistencies were also highly unreliable: some were too greasy, others too dry. The colors I found at the drugstore, were surprisingly quite good, and some of the textures were smooth without being greasy or dry. The same is true for blushers; drugstore blushers are every bit as wonderful as department store blushers and the price difference is almost absurd. Even the new cream-to-powder blushes are available at the drugstore and they are just as reliable as the ones you'll buy at the cosmetics counter.

In terms of skin care, I can't encourage you strongly enough to avoid wasting money on expensive department store skin care items. There is no reason in the world to believe that the cosmetics counter products are any better for your skin than those you can purchase at the drugstore. Read the ingredient labels and you'll know that this is true. I know this is hard to swallow. After all, how could a $100 wrinkle cream be as good for your face as a $5 cream? But test this one out for yourself: Use an expensive skin cream on one side of your face, and use one or two of my inexpensive suggestions (see Chapter Seven) on the other side. I will be surprised if you notice any difference at all.

CHAPTER FOUR

Facing the Truth About Skin Care

SKIN CARE UPDATE

I wrote extensively about the entire subject of skin care and skin care routines in both of my *Blue Eyeshadow* books. Here I will review the skin care routine I recommend most often and answer the questions I am asked most frequently. In Chapter Seven I will evaluate many of the specific skin care products that are now being sold by the major cosmetics companies.

Let me state from the beginning that there are no perfect skin care products: Quality comes down to what works for you and not what is the most expensive or reputedly the "best" product. I have talked to hundreds of women who have jumped from one expensive skin care line to another in a desperate search for the perfect routine. I will give you the basics of a good skin care routine and tell you what I think works. I will expose the myths at every opportunity, but as usual, you and your skin will make the final decision. Every woman needs to learn to recognize what her skin and common sense are telling her.

Over the years I have received numerous letters and phone calls from people who sell skin care products via home marketing programs. They call wanting me to give them an honest evaluation of the products they are selling. The basic merchandising premise they all share is the claim of authenticity. Almost every time, a similar story accompanies each line of products: a chemist, physician, pharmacist, dermatologist, makeup artist, actress or actor, cancer specialist (and who knows who else?) has formulated some "remarkable, unprecedented skin care product or products that can do what others can't do for your skin." In each case, the doctor or "specialist" in these stories say they have formulated products for a client or patient suffering terribly from some skin problem; after using the product, the patient's skin sprang back to life! Another thing these products have in common is a lack of unique ingredients. I have yet to see one that contains anything unusual or unique. They are all made from the same ingredients you would find in other moisturizers and other skin care products on the market, but each has its own intriguing marketing twist to make it sound like you're truly getting something remarkable.

Here are the skin care basics: a cleanser; an exfoliating product, such as a scrub; a disinfectant if you have blemishes; a moisturizer if you have dry skin; and a more emollient night cream, but only if you have extremely dry skin. You will find these basic products in various forms and combinations in almost every skin care line. Yet we agonize over which product or which company has developed the secret to procuring a peaches-and-cream complexion; we expect that the perfect combination of products will make us look like the models in the magazines and on television. I do not suggest for one moment that some benefit cannot be gained from the use of skin care products; it's just that perfect skin — that carrot of hope you'll find dangled in the form of beautiful, over-priced containers and jars — is not possible.

What is and isn't possible when it comes to your skin? I'm glad you asked. Here's the good news and the bad:

✔ A simple, gentle skin care routine will keep your skin looking its best, but it won't cure acne or get rid of wrinkles.

✔ It doesn't have to cost a lot to achieve a nice complexion. Because there are more similarities between skin care products than differences, spending less won't hurt your skin, and spending more won't necessarily help it.

✔ If you are exposed to the sun, even a little, your skin will wrinkle and there are no cosmetic products that can change that. There is no such thing as careful tanning, safe tanning or wrinkle-proof tanning. Using a suntan lotion with an SPF of 15 or greater is the only way to avoid premature wrinkling.

✔ Even the most perfect skin will get a blemish on occasion. If you tend to breakout, you will breakout, and if you tend to have oily skin, you will have oily skin. If you try to "dry up" blemishes or dry up the oil on your skin, all you will have is dried-up skin that is still oily (as anyone with this skin-type knows).

✓ Ironically, a great number of skin care problems are caused by the skin care products women use most frequently to prevent them. Many problems are caused by allergic reactions or by using products that are too irritating, too drying or too thick and creamy.

✓ Using too many moisturizers or moisturizers that are too emollient can cause whiteheads and blackheads.

✓ Skin may become inflamed, dry and blemished if you use too many scrubs at the same time — for example, a granular cleanser and loofah, or a washcloth and an abrasive scrub, or a scrub and an astringent or toner, one after the other. If you use the wrong products or too many products on your face at the same time, you are likely to develop skin irritations or breakouts.

✓ Harsh soaps and cleansers (even some that claim they are gentle) can cause the skin to become too dry. Washing with a bar soap or harsh cleanser will leave your face feeling tight and dry and will cause you to have dry skin. Then you'll use more moisturizer than you otherwise would have needed; in fact, if not for the harsh cleanser you might not have needed a moisturizer at all. Furthermore, you risk ending up with clogged pores.

✓ Many cleansers that claim they are water-soluble are really too greasy to rinse off completely; they, too, can cause clogged pores.

✓ In general, the fewer products you use on your skin, the better for your skin. The more you use the greater your chances of allergic reactions, cosmetic acne and irritation.

✓ There is no credible reason to use different moisturizers on your body then you do on your face. If one moisturizer takes care of dry skin on your legs, it will most probably do a great job of taking care of the dry skin on your face.

✓ It's problematic to seek skin care products based on your skin type. More often than not, your skin type is not what you think it is. Possibly your skin type has been created by the products you are already using: Soap can severely dry the skin, or a wrinkle cream can clog pores and cause blemishes. Thus, using more products would only make matters worse, not better. Furthermore the wrong recommendations are often made for a particular skin condition. For example, a woman who feels she has combination or oily skin may find herself being sold a scrub product and a toner that contains alcohol, to be used one after the other on a daily basis. This can be so irritating that it causes her skin to breakout even more or become even more dry. To counter the irritation, she will be sold moisturizers to use on the areas that have become dry, and this can further clog her pores.

✓ The most coveted skin is that with no visible pores, but that skin type doesn't come in a bottle. There are no products available anywhere that can close pores for any longer than a few minutes.

✓ Teenagers are not the only ones who have acne. Women in their thirties are among the largest group to get acne. Not everyone who has acne as a teenager will grow out of it, and if you had clear skin as a teenager it doesn't mean that you won't get acne later in life.

✓ A myth that has hung around the world of cosmetics and beauty long enough is that dry skin ages faster than oily skin. This is not true. Lighter or fair skin tones age faster than darker skin tones. If you don't include a sunscreen with an SPF of 15 or greater, even if you lather on creams and lotions, your skin will still wrinkle. Enough said.

✓ One of the best ways to deal with extremely dry skin is to find a gentle skin care routine. Do not use anything on your face that is drying — washcloths, tissues, harsh scrubs, hot water, dry saunas, toners or fresheners that contain alcohol or other drying ingredients.

✓ The best way to calm down oily skin is to use a gentle skin care routine. Irritation causes an increase in oil production, which clogs the pores, which in turn may cause blackheads. The next step is to avoid products that contain ingredients that can clog pores. As a general rule, use a scrub product at least once a day for oily skin and every other day for drier skin. The final step: Gently squeeze the blackhead to remove it.

✓ Oil-free moisturizers are a curious group of products. They are usually sold to acne-prone women with dry skin, combination skin or those who are worried about their skin wrinkling if they don't use a moisturizer of some kind. There are three fallacies involved with this type of product: 1) Oil-free moisturizers (and all oil-free products, for that matter) usually exclude heavy emollients from their ingredient list, but these are not the only ingredients that can cause flare-up of acne or blackheads. I have used many oil-free products that have caused my skin to break-out; 2) If you have oily skin with dry patches, the reason can often be traced to the skin care products you are using to cleanse your face — soaps, detergent cleansers, astringents, toners, harsh scrubs, over-scrubbing and clay masks can all make oily skin dry and if you stop using them you may eliminate your dry skin problems; 3) If you have oily skin and no dry patches, then use of a moisturizer of any kind is a waste of money. When you have your own built-in moisturizer, why buy someone else's? As you now know, neither moisturizers or nor wrinkle creams can stop or prevent wrinkling.

When should you consider using an oil-free moisturizer? Only if your skin is oily and truly dry in patches and the dryness isn't caused by other skin care products you may be using. It is also a good idea to try oil-free moisturizers if you know that your skin reacts to oils and other ingredients included in moisturizers designed for normal or combination skin types.

MY BASIC SKIN CARE ROUTINE

This is a condensed version of what I recommend in my *Blue Eyeshadow Should Be Illegal* books:

Step 1: Even at night, when you're removing makeup, always wash your face with a water-soluble cleanser that rinses off completely and doesn't irritate the eyes. Your eye makeup should come off with the same water-soluble cleanser that cleans your face. It shouldn't be necessary to use an extra product to wipe across the eye, pulling the skin and eyelashes unnecessarily. (Wiping off makeup in general is never good for the skin; the wiping pulls at the skin and a tissue or washcloth can irritate it.) The product I recommend for cleansing all skin types is Cetaphil lotion, available at a reasonable price in most drugstores. It is neither greasy nor drying and has no coloring agents or fragrance. I will review other cleansers in Chapter Seven, but for cost and efficiency, Cetaphil is still one of the best I've found.

Step 2: Use only tepid to slightly warm water only. Hot water burns the skin, and cold water shocks it.

Step 3A: If your skin is oily and tends to breakout, after you've rinsed off the Cetaphil Lotion and, while the face is still wet, pour a handful of baking soda into the palm of your hand. Add a small amount of water to the baking soda to create a paste. Gently massage the entire face with this paste, and then rinse generously with tepid water. Be extra careful not to get carried away: Over-scrubbing can cause more problems than it solves. The operative word for all skin care is "gentle."

Step 3B: If you have combination skin, follow Step 3A, but massage only those areas that tend to breakout, and avoid the areas that are dry.

Step 3C: If you have normal skin, follow Step 3A, but only three or four times a week.

Step 3D: If you have dry skin, rinse off the Cetaphil lotion completely and, while the face is still wet, pour about a tablespoon of baking soda into the palm of your hand. Add a generous amount of Cetaphil and a small amount of water. Use this paste as a very light, gentle scrub for your face, but don't get carried away. Rinse generously with tepid water. Repeat only three times a week.

Step 3E: If you have extremely dry skin, follow step 3D, but use more Cetaphil than baking soda in your mixture and be very, very, gentle when massaging the face. Repeat only twice a week.

Step 4: The time to gently squeeze any blackheads or blemishes is after your face is completely cleansed. NEVER, absolutely NEVER over-squeeze. If the blemish does not respond easily, stop and leave it alone. Squeezing in and of itself does not cause problems on the face; in fact it is one of the best ways to clean out the skin. The problems occur when you massacre the skin by squeezing to the point where you create scabs and sores on the face.

Step 5A: When the face is completely rinsed and dried and you've finished any squeezing that you need to do, take a cotton ball soaked in 3 percent hydrogen peroxide and go over those areas that breakout. Hydrogen peroxide works as a disinfectant and will bleach the discoloration of blackheads. Do not use this step if you don't breakout. You can use the 3 percent hydrogen peroxide in place of an astringent or toner once or twice a day.

Step 5B: If you have normal to dry skin that does not breakout, rinse your face completely and go over the face with a skin freshener that does not contain alcohol. Although I generally think of this as an unnecessary step, many women feel it is important. Some of the products I recommend are: Lancome's Tonique Douceur, Chanel's Lotion Douce, L'Oreal's

Floral Tonic, Ultima II's CHR Extraordinary Gentle Clarifier, Physicians Formula's Gentle Refreshing Toner and Clinique's Alcohol-Free Clarifiier. None of these contains irritants such as alcohol or acetone. All of them can impart a pleasant sensation to the face, but for the most part they are not worth the exorbitant price tag (especially when you consider the total cost of their basic ingredients: water, glycerin, polypropylene glycol, dimethicone copolyol and some herb extracts). Fresheners are neither essential nor harmful, so long as they do not contain ingredients that can irritate the skin.

Step 5C: If your skin is extremely oily or breaks out frequently, you may consider trying a facial mask of plain Phillip's Milk of Magnesia. Milk of Magnesia is a mixture of magnesium and water. Magnesium is a good disinfectant, and it can absorb oil. The clay masks you find on the market for oily skin have no disinfecting properties, and their ingredients cannot absorb oil as well as magnesium. Your skin type and reaction to the mask will determine how often you can use it. Those with severely oily skin, may use it every day; those with slightly oily skin should only need to use it once a week.

Step 6: If you do not have dry skin, you do not need a moisturizer. You may want to wear a moisturizing sunscreen during the day to protect your face from the damaging rays of the sun, however. A face smothered with lotions and wrinkle creams will not age any differently from one on which no creams and lotions have been used.

Step 7: If you have dry skin, or dry to normal skin, apply a light lotion-type moisturizer to your face over a light layer of water and allow it to absorb into the skin rather than rubbing it into the skin. My favorite moisturizers are Lubriderm (fragrance-free only), Nutraderm, Eucerin and Nivea. These are some of the best and most reasonably priced moisturizers on the market. Try these before you venture into the higher priced brands. For areas on the face that are more dry than others, you may want to use a thicker more emollient-type moisturizer, but just over those areas and just at night. A pure oil can do the same thing, but a cream may feel better and absorb more readily.

Step 8: If you have severely dry skin, you may want to consult a dermatologist.

Step 9: If you have severe acne, consult your dermatologist about the use of Accutane. This is a serious, expensive drug to use, but its success rate in curing chronic acne is remarkable.

RETIN-A UPDATE

There is little controversy over the fact that Retin-A thins the outer layer of skin and, to some extent, improves the appearance of sun-damaged skin. There is also some inconclusive evidence that Retin-A may someday prove useful as a first step in combating some forms of skin cancer. What is more controversial, and still not widely accepted, is how much change actually takes place and whether or not Retin-A can stimulate the growth of collagen and elastin in the lower layers of skin.

Despite the unknowns, Retin-A is here to stay: The FDA is expected to approve Retin-A for use as an anti-photoaging (anti-sun-damaging) prescription drug. That prospect doesn't change anything for the consumer; it simply gives Johnson & Johnson more outlets to market Retin-A. Already Retin-A, as an FDA-approved acne treatment, can be prescribed for anything a dermatologist or physician deems necessary; the only restriction is that Johnson & Johnson can't market the drug specifically as a wrinkle cream. Obviously, there are immense loop-holes in that restriction, or every woman and her sister wouldn't think of Retin-A as a wrinkle cream.

When it comes to Retin-A, don't believe any wild claims. Retin-A is not a *cure* for wrinkles, and it does not take the place of staying out of the sun or getting a face-lift. But there are practical benefits that can be gained from using Retin-A: In some women it may result in rosier, smoother skin, diminished acne lesions, a reduction in the amount of wrinkles, or a combination of all the above. Of the people I interviewed, including dermatologists, nurses who worked for dermatologists, and women who have used Retin-A for an extended period of time, nearly all reported positive results. None felt that their skin was as wrinkle-free as perhaps Johnson & Johnson would like us to believe, and a large number said they saw no difference in their wrinkles but thought their skin appeared smoother. When I began using Retin-A I felt my skin was smoother and somewhat rosier, and I saw a small change in the appearance of the wrinkles around my eyes but little to no change on my forehead. Bottom line: Retin-A may be worth a try if you are over 30 and have sun-damaged skin.

In *Blue Eyeshadow Should Still Be Illegal*, I wrote extensively about how to use Retin-A and what you should expect during the first three to six months of use. Here are some of those points:

✓ You cannot tan after you start using Retin-A: 1) because the skin is more sensitive to sunlight while you are using the drug and is therefore more subject to serious sunburn; and 2) because tanning will negate any positive effects you were hoping to gain from using Retin-A.

✓ Please remember that the first thing Retin-A does to the skin is irritate it. If you use any other irritant on the skin at the same time, you will exacerbate the initial negative side effects of the drug. You must eliminate all of the following from your skin care routine during the first months of using Retin-A: washcloths, hot water, cold water, all astringents, toners, fresheners, clarifying lotions, refining lotions and the like, scrubs, facial masks, bar soaps, skin care products that contain fragrance or strong preservatives, saunas, steam rooms, and any and all products that contain alcohol. It is essential you continue to use a fragrance-free moisturizer.

✓ Many of the studies you will read about Retin-A in the media or in medical journals may be sponsored by Johnson & Johnson, the manufacturer of Retin-A. Obviously, Johnson & Johnson have a vested interest in proving that Retin-A is, indeed, a medical treatment for wrinkles.

✓ Do not think of Retin-A as a cosmetic. Do not borrow a tube of it from a friend or ask your children's pediatrician or your gynecologist for a prescription. Although I disagree with some of the things dermatologists recommend for skin care, I believe that they are the best source for Retin-A therapy.

✓ If you want Retin-A to work, you must use it regularly. To sustain the results, you need to continue using it for the rest of your life. The changes that take place on the skin are said not to be permanent. Initial studies seem to indicate that once you stop using the product, the skin slowly reverts to it's original condition — more or less. Using something forever is a scary proposition and a tremendous commitment. For me, however, the difference I see on my skin is positive enough to warrant the long-term relationship.

"Cosmetics are used by teenage girls to make them look older sooner, and by their mothers to make them look younger longer."

CHAPTER 5

Makeup Update

WHAT'S NEW AT THE COSMETICS COUNTER

The cosmetics counters are an endless source of amazement for me. As I've said before, the vast selection of products is nothing less than astounding. Sometimes the stunning new displays are just recycled colors with new packaging and new names. Other times there are new products that either make the application of makeup easier, or sometimes more difficult. Those of you who shopped for makeup in the 1970s must recall seeing fat eyeliner pencils? I complained about them at length in those days and would never have recommended them to anyone. Fat eyeliner pencils were hard, if not impossible, to sharpen, they were greasy and smudged too easily, and because it was hard to keep a point in place, the application to the eye of a thin stretch of color was almost impossible. It took a while, but fat eyeliner pencils have become a thing of the past. You can't sell women something that doesn't work for too long, because ultimately they do catch on and won't tolerate it anymore.

Well, this is 1991 and there is a new procession of products for your consideration. Most are variations on the same old theme with a few interesting twists, but it is fair to say that there really isn't anything new under the sun. The basics of getting your makeup on haven't changed one bit: foundation, concealer, finishing powder (loose or pressed), blush, eyeshadows, eyeliner, brow pencil, lipliner and lipstick are still what it takes. I guess the cliché applies: The more things change, the more they stay the same. The following is a list of the "new" basic makeup products you will find at the cosmetics counter:

FOUNDATIONS: Almost every cosmetics line has at least four different types of makeup base, and many have five or six. This overwhelming assortment breaks down into the following general categories: an oil-free liquid foundation for oily skin, a water-based liquid foundation for normal to dry skin, a water-based liquid foundation with extra emollients or thicker coverage for dry skin, a cream powder compact foundation that goes on like a cream but dries to a powder finish, and traditional cream foundation that either comes in a stick or in a compact for extremely dry skin.

The newest product is the cream-to-powder compact foundation. This interesting product goes on smooth and creamy, providing light to medium coverage. The texture of these products is lovely. Almost every cosmetics line from the department store to the drugstore has one of these. The only negative thing is that this product works best on normal skin types. Dry skin can look chalky and parched with this type of foundation and oily skin sometimes absorbs the powder into the pores and looks dotted. Borghese makes an interesting variation on this theme; their cream powder foundation is a liquid in a compact, but it can be somewhat messy to use. It is an excellent product, and for those with normal to slightly oily skin, this foundation is worth checking out.

Another type of foundation that has been around for a short period of time is an oil-free foundation that is half glycerin and half talc. This makes for an interesting suspension of color in a slippery liquid that feels wet on the face when it's applied and dries to become a normal-looking foundation. If you are careful, you can get an extremely sheer finish with this product. My experience is that this is a tricky foundation to use. The liquid is somewhat hard to control and it may take awhile to grow accustomed to the feel of the glycerin on the skin. Another potential problem is the glycerin content; though glycerin in small amounts is not usually a problem, when it is a large percentage of the product it can be an irritant. Both Prescriptives and Adrien Arpel carry this type of foundation and I had an allergic reaction to both of them.

Today, there is a wide selection of oil-free foundations. They seem to be popping up all over. Ultima II has two new foundations that are oil-free and one is recommended for dry skin. Fashion Fair, Revlon (drugstore), Clinique and Charles of the Ritz all have more than one oil-free foundation. Most of the new oil-free foundations I've tested are really quite excellent, with light textures that give beautiful coverage. The only ones I do not recommend are those that contain alcohol, like the Pore Minimizer by Clinique.

CONCEALERS: From the considerable new array of concealers on the market you would think that none of us would have a dark circle to worry about. Unfortunately, in spite of this whopping selection of shades and consistencies, most of the colors are either too dark, too orange, too rose, too pink, too greasy (filling in the lines around the eye), too dry, too thick, or too thin. I can understand the different textures — something for every preference — but why the strange assortment of shades is beyond me. There is no way a concealer that is darker than your foundation, or darker than your skin tone or has orange or pink tones can make any dark area lighter. If you want to lighten something, you have to put a light color on it — something that matches the foundation or, at the very least, won't darken the color of the foundation. Concealers in other than a neutral tone will alter the shade of the foundation around the eye; you will get an odd color wherever the concealer and the foundation merge. I recommend concealers in neutral tones that are much lighter than the foundation, and there are plenty of those on the market. The concept is that the light undereye concealer goes on first, the foundation blends over it (so there are no edges where they join) and thus makes the foundation look lighter under the eye.

FINISHING POWDERS: I guess it isn't surprising that a product as simple and basic as pressed and loose powder can end up with as much marketing hype as any wrinkle cream or skin treatment. The best thing that has happened to "setting" or "finishing" powders is that there is a wider range of color choices than ever before and the selection of consistencies ranges from silky to sheer. The negative things are the claims that accompany the products. Basically all pressed and loose powders are either talc, wheat or cornstarch, zinc stearate and nylon-12 or some combination thereof. Talc is the mainstay, though there are talc free powders, which are not any better or worse on the skin than those powders with talc. There is absolutely no reason to spend a lot of money on pressed or loose powders.

BLUSHES: Almost every cosmetic line now carries the new cream powder blushes. These are similar, if not identical to cream powder foundations. They are wonderful for those who have normal to oily skin. Hard edges are a thing of the past once you learn how to apply cream powder blushes, although they can be a bit tricky to apply. Borghese makes a liquid version of the cream to powder blush. It works very well over normal to oily skin.

EYESHADOWS: I have spoken out for over eight years about the problems of wearing shiny eyeshadows, but it has been almost impossible to find attractive matte shades. Two of the major reasons for avoiding shiny eyeshadows are that they make the skin on the lid look wrinkly and they are as inappropriate for daytime as would be a sequinned evening gown. Yet the cosmetics industry has continued to maintain its abundant selection of iridescent colors. In the meantime consumers have learned that shiny eyeshadows don't look great, we've noticed that models in the magazines or on ads and brochures selling makeup aren't wearing shiny eyeshadows, and it is becoming common knowledge that flat eyeshadows go on more evenly and smoothly. Slowly but surely many cosmetics lines have seen the light. There is now, more then ever before, a wonderful variety of matte eyeshadow colors. I have listed the specific shades in Chapter Six. You will be surprised, however, how many product lines are still lagging behind. I predict it will be only a matter of time before shiny eyeshadows are hard to find and matte colors are the predominant selections available at the cosmetics counters and on the drugstore makeup racks.

LIPSTICKS: The least amount of change in makeup has taken place with lipstick. Women still prefer a creamy texture to a dry or greasy feel on the mouth. Not that the cosmetics companies have stopped producing greasy lipsticks, but there remain only a handful of color choices, compared to a huge array of creamy textured lipsticks. Matte colors are becoming more and more popular as cosmetics companies try to deal with the problem of lip color bleeding or feathering into the lines around the mouth. Many lines have introduced lipsticks that contain powder (usually talc or kaolin), or somewhat creamy powders which supposedly prevent bleeding or feathering into the lines around the mouth. But I have found that lipsticks that contain powder or clay dry out the lips and make them look chapped and parched and none of them prevented lipstick from feathering into the lines around my mouth. There are a few products that are designed specifically to keep lipstick from feathering, and some of them work like miracles and others are a waste of money. See Chapter Eight for my recommendations.

LIP PENCILS: There are a handful of gimmicky lip-lining products around, such as waterproof lip pencils (if having red lips while swimming is important to you), lip pencils that incorporate a lip brush at one end of the pencil, and automatic pencils that conveniently eliminate sharpening. All of these pencils, regardless of their price tag, do essentially the same job. There is little to no difference between a $3 lip pencil and a $22 lip pencil, so spending more dollars here will not improve the look of your mouth.

EYE PENCILS: If you thought the task of selecting an eyeliner was an easy one, guess again. The vast number of options for lining the eye is literally astounding: liquid liners in a tube, thin eye pencils, fat eye pencils, automatic eye pencils, eye pencils designed like a felt-tip pen, pencils that don't have to be sharpened because the material around the tip peels away, pencils with sponges at one end, pencils with a powder eyeshadow and applicator at one end, and waterproof eye pencils for those who want their eyes to stay lined while they jog in the rain. The different textures produce a wide assortment of looks, from subtle to exotic. Liquid liners or felt-tip pen eyeliners tend to create a more dramatic, obvious lined look, while thin pencils or automatic pencils can create either a soft or a more obvious lined look. Many pencils come packaged with a sponge tip at one end for blending (to soften the line) or to use for shading at the back corner of the eye. Here is yet another area where it doesn't make much sense to spend a lot of money, since there is little difference between brands, but again the automatic pencils that don't require sharpening are extremely convenient.

EYEBROW PENCILS: Eyebrows that look drawn on with a pencil are dated — like pancake makeup or false eyelashes — but many women still have them. Alternatives have come along over the years, like eyebrow powders, yet they have never really replaced using a brow pencil to fill in sparse or nonexistent eyebrows. The major difference in eyebrow pencils these days is that the good ones have a drier texture; the brows they create look less greasy and obvious than they used to. Some brow pencils come with a brush at one end, thus encouraging the user to comb through the line and soften it once the color has been drawn into place. The latest product showing up at the cosmetics counters is a brow gel with color. These mascara-looking products are brushed on through the brow much like a mascara is brushed on through the eyelashes, to make the existing brow hair look fuller and darker. This innovation is a welcome addition for those women who want a fuller-looking brow without the artificial appearance a pencil can create.

MASCARAS: This is one area of makeup that has always fascinated and frustrated me. If I wear nothing else, I wear mascara, lipstick, and a little blush. I might even omit the lipstick and the blush, or my lipstick might wear off by the second cup of coffee and the blush be history by my second phone conversation, but I would not omit the mascara, nor would I tolerate its wearing off. A good mascara goes on fast and easily and doesn't flake, smudge, wear off or clump. So what's the frustration? Finding a mascara that doesn't do any of the things I've just mentioned above. The only mascaras I did not test during my research are waterproof mascaras. For daytime or evening wear, waterproof mascaras are no more reliable than water-soluble mascaras. Both water-soluble and waterproof mascaras will smudge and smear if your eyes tend to get oily during the day or if you wear a moisturizer or a moisture-rich foundation. Waterproof mascaras are also hard on the lashes because they can only be removed with a greasy cleanser that is wiped off. Such wiping can easily pull out delicate lashes. But don't worry, I have found a great assortment of water-soluble mascaras to recommend, and you will find them all in Chapter Six.

HAS MAKEUP FASHION CHANGED?

The concept of fashion makeup, as in "What's the latest fashion makeup trend?" or "What direction is fashion makeup taking nowadays?" always bothers me. I think it brings out the part of me that resents being told what to do. Why should Madison Avenue or fashion designers or makeup designers dictate what I should put on when I get up in the morning or go out in the evening? Besides, there is such a voluminous assortment of products and colors at the cosmetics counters and drugstores that you can literally put together any look your heart desires. Yet, there is a definite "direction" that exists and binds together the various fashion makeup statements. Whether or not you want to follow the trend is totally up to you. My suggestion is that being "fashionable" is not the worst thing you can do. Beehive hairdos, Nehru jackets and go-go boots, and — more to the subject at hand — false eyelashes, lips outlined in brown, and blue eyeshadow might have looked great back when, but today they look unquestionably out of place. Suffice it to say that an attractive, fashionable makeup application is an important part of any woman's appearance. Besides, fashion makeup nowadays is easier and less obtrusive than ever before.

What is fashionable? Soft makeup that is played down not up. I see this theme repeated on magazine covers month after month. Even the

Cosmo woman, with her ever deepening cleavage and provocative posturing, wears neutral eyeshadows and eyeliner and soft blush, with no vivid colors to be seen anywhere. Her sensual appearance comes from the definition around the eyes and the exaggerated full mouth, not from intensely bright eyeshadow or other makeup colors. The idea is not to have the makeup take control of your face and radically alter it, but for makeup to be subtle, soft and flattering.

I hope we will never see a return of the before-and-after makeup ads. We all know makeup can be a powerful fashion tool; it just doesn't have to be the tool by which we define our own standard of beauty. More and more I find women drawn to a subdued, less colorful makeup fashion statement. The increased availability of matte eyeshadows, the emphasis on the different ways to line the eyes and color the mouth, all are evidence that women are more interested in playing up their features instead of over-coloring them. Even the foundation shades are more and more neutral. It used to be difficult to find foundations that weren't overly pink, peach, rose or orange; now the color selections are more in line with actual skin tones of ivory, beige, tan, bronze and ebony. Whether or not the cosmetics companies are ready to admit it 100 percent, the sales of foundations with overtones of pink, peach, rose and orange are decreasing rapidly.

Having encouraged you to follow in the same direction that makeup fashion is currently taking, I certainly don't want to see the fashion revert to a more obvious makeup look. It is important to mention that the cosmetics companies in a struggle to gain control over how we buy makeup and to increase sales, will at times try to market more explicit makeup look. It is up to us to make sure we don't fall for it. Does this mean we have control over fashion? No, not exactly. Sometimes fashion is part of a greater picture than we have control over. But nowadays, more often than not, if we don't buy what they're selling, the fashion designers go out of business. So, in a rather major way we have control over what's fashionable. Designers have to earn a living too, and if we don't get sucked into doing what feels uncomfortable, they won't resell it to us next year. The natural, less madeup look has been around for awhile now; let's make sure it stays.

FOR WOMEN OF COLOR

Fifteen years ago, when I was first establishing myself as a makeup artist in Washington, D.C., I had the opportunity to do the makeup for a beauty contest for African-American women. I spent an entire week trying to find lipsticks, eyeshadows, foundations and blushes that would be suitable for this large a group of African-American women. At the time, suitable products were scarce; even the cosmetics lines designed for women of color had foundations that were too orange and greasy, the lipsticks were all too dark, bordering on black, and there were virtually no eyeshadows intense enough for very dark skin tones. If it was difficult for me as a makeup artist, imagine how frustrating it was for the women who needed makeup products that would suit their deeper skin color.

How times have changed! Almost all lines now carry makeup products for women of color, and the color selections are superior. Foundations for African-American women are no longer automatically greasy, and the orange tint is greatly reduced or almost nonexistent. Lipstick colors come in a wide range of shades, taking into consideration that not all African-American women want dark-colored lips. Among the best of the improvements is that the darker shades of blush are no longer grainy and dry; most are smooth and silky and go on beautifully.

For African-American women and other women of color, there are many options available in several of the traditional cosmetics lines and particularly the cosmetics lines designed specifically for darker skin tones. The widest selection possible is to be found at the Fashion Fair and Flory Roberts counters, particularly for lipsticks, foundations, blushes and concealing creams. There is still a problem of shiny eyeshadows to be dealt with and some of the lipsticks designed for women of color tend toward the greasy side, but those are minor problems in comparison to how extensive they used to be. A major problem for African-American women, however, is that many of the leading cosmetics lines, particularly those at drugstores, still have a small selection of foundations, powders and concealers for darker skin tones. The situation is changing at a surprisingly slow pace given the number of African-American female consumers. The cosmetics companies will have to catch up eventually or be left in the dust.

CHOOSING WHAT LOOKS GOOD ON YOU

I would need to see you personally in order to help you evaluate how something looks on you. After all, if you're blonde and fair-skinned, a soft bronze lipstick might look beautiful on you; but if your blonde hair comes from a bottle and you have sallow skin, a bronze lipstick could make you look sick. If you have vibrant red hair and classic white skin, a magenta lipstick or pink eyeshadow could make your face look inflamed and swollen. Once you've established what colors look best on you, there is a broad spectrum of makeup color schemes, and selecting from them is not your only dilemma: You must also consider your own lifestyle, the colors in your wardrobe, the look you want to achieve at work and at play, how much makeup you feel comfortable wearing and what is an appropriate amount of makeup for each occasion. All of these factors should influence what makeup shades you choose to wear.

There is also the question of taste, individuality and the degree of effort you're willing to expend on your looks. Besides, if we have a very specific notion of what makes us look good and what works for us, there is almost nothing anyone can do to change that opinion. Nothing is as difficult for women as the challenge of self-objectivity. One of the most poignant portrayals of this was shown in the movie *Working Girl* with Melanie Griffith and Sigourney Weaver. Weaver's character plays a successful business woman, and Griffith's character is her over-madeup, rather gauche assistant who desperately wants to move ahead in her career. When the assistant finally finds the means to her end, part of the game-plan involves acquiring a more sophisticated hairdo and wardrobe and more subtle, less obvious makeup. The movie reflects that how we look affects the way others see us. Although it's nice to "do your own thing," it's best to do it on your day off. I know it's hard to change — people I work with show me all the time:

I had a long standing client who always asked me for recommendations about her makeup, and every time she asked, I would tell her to stop wearing brown lipstick and brown blush. She insisted that they were the only colors that looked good on her. As far as she was concerned, when I said "no brown," she thought I was telling her to wear flaming red. Of course, there are a great many colors that exist between red and brown, but Joyce couldn't see that. I finally decided to send her a couple of lipsticks and blushes that I thought would look great on her along with a note that said, "Trust me!" A short while later, I ran into Joyce in a local department store — she was wearing the new lipstick and blush. I almost said "I told you so," but after we said hello, I told her how good she looked and changed the subject.

I started doing Estee's makeup when she was 16. Now she's in her early twenties and I've noticed she started lining her lower lashes with a heavy black liquid liner that cracks and peels by the end of the day. No matter how often I tell her that the result is messy and unattractive, she refuses to change her product. She insists that if she lines with a powder as I recommend, she won't look good and the liner won't last. The last time I saw her, I gave her one of those new felt-tip lining pens that place a thinner liquid line along the eyelashes and that don't crack or peel. I've just received a note from Estee thanking me for the new eyeliner and saying that she would never doubt my suggestions again.

I have an exuberant friend whom I often see at my hairdresser's. Every time I see Marta, she is wearing the wrong foundation color. There is always a visible line at her jaw. She is a very observant woman, and when she sees me glancing at her neck (it's hard for me not to), she quickly rubs her jaw and hastily explains what a hurry she was in that morning and how she just threw herself together. From time to time I've said to her that she could blend all day and her foundation would still be the wrong color. What it boils down to is that she just hates her skin and wishes it were tan and flawless, but it's not. She continues to use heavy foundations that make her skin look darker, and the result is the inevitable line at her jaw or along her neck and collar. I guess you can't win them all.

Jennifer works at a cosmetics counter where I shop quite a bit. She is a show-stopper. She carries herself with grace and confidence and dresses immaculately. She is someone who would look good in mud. Yet she makes mistakes with makeup I just can't understand. She already has thick dark lashes, but she thickens them further with mascara until they resemble bars across a window, giving her kind of a strained surprised look. She also matches her eyeshadow to whatever outfit she's wearing: lavender skirt, lavender shadow; blue blouse, blue eyeshadow; green jacket, green eyeshadow. The shadows always look too obvious. I decided to stretch our professional relationship and asked her if I could suggest a different eye design. She agreed and we had a great time while I applied more neutral shades of eyeshadow, softer eyeliner and mascara — she was surprised at the results. I pointed out to her that it was more fashionable to wear soft, neutral eyeshadow colors and pastel lip and blush colors that are in a similar color tone to her wardrobe. Several weeks later I saw her wearing the same eye design I had created for her, and I knew she'd been convinced.

To be perfectly honest, of late I've noticed that my ego is getting in the way of how I apply my own makeup. Blush colors have gotten much softer over the past several years, but I have a tendency to wear vivid blush colors as I do when I appear on television, even when I'm dressing only for a business meeting. My close friend Julie asked me why I didn't tone down the amount of blush I wear. I agreed that I was being heavy-handed and, although I know that I have a tendency to be too enthusiastic with my blush, I was having trouble cutting back. I feel so pale when I don't look the way I'm used to looking. Like everybody, I'm accustomed to seeing a certain face in the mirror, and so it is hard to change, even though I know better. When I started writing this book and began playing with hundreds of products, I finally found a sheer-looking blush that I really like on me. It took awhile, but better late than never.

THE COSMETICS INDUSTRY:
WHERE IT'S BEEN AND WHERE IT'S GOING

For those of us over 30, there was a time when we weren't booming. There was a time when we were babies, children, teenagers and young adults. Throughout the decades, to some degree or another, we spent each year dealing with what it meant to be women in this complex world. Regardless of whatever else was going on in our lives, the cosmetics industry was right there, every step of the way, and reckoning with them and our consumer impulses has been a long, arduous and endless task.

Even when I was little, I knew that it was important to be attractive. I also learned from early on that it took a great deal of time and energy to look beautiful. I remember sitting on the edge of the bathtub watching my mother paint her lips red and color her eyelids with shades of blue and lavender. I can clearly see her taking out her compact during the day and fixing her lipstick or powdering her nose in the evening. At night I was mesmerized by her bedtime ritual of smearing on cold cream. All the colors that were neatly in place only moments before swirled and streaked together. Using tissue after tissue, Mom wiped, methodically, until the gooey mess was gone. When the cream was entirely removed, a slick, filmy appearance was left behind that made the skin on her face look shiny and moist. To finish the process she would place clips in her hair, secure a net over the silvery array, and go to sleep. Night after night, that production relayed powerful information for a little girl to assimilate. I understood from a very early age that beauty was not only complicated; it wasn't even pretty.

When I became a teenager, and the hormones were flowing through my body and out my ears, being beautiful was still a struggle. But by the 1960s and the early 1970s, the routine had changed. Wavy, curly hair was no longer popular, so we tortured our locks on ironing boards or with orange juice cans used as rollers to discipline unfashionably curly hair into perfectly straight lines. Of course, if it started to rain or an ounce of humidity appeared in the air, the tenacity of the natural curl won out. Regarding makeup, we had two choices: to place a white highlighter under the eyebrow, a stripe of brown across the crease and a shade of blue on the lid; or to do nothing at all à la the "natural look." Makeup was artificial, yet this was the era of the "flower child." What a double message: Not wearing makeup meant looking beautiful "naturally," but the majority of us found that impossible to accept when we looked in the mirror. So, many of us searched for "natural" makeup, products that would give our faces the color we thought was missing. When it came to skin care, we exhausted ourselves with facials, acne gels, tubes of Clearasil and bottles of astringents. I could never wash my face enough. If it hurt, I thought my skin would improve. Of course, nothing I did ever really helped. Just as my hair never stayed straight, my face never stayed clear.

The middle and late 1970s was a time for experimentation. We painted Twiggy lashes under the lower eyelashes, etched plastic eyeliner on the lids, drew brown lipliner around our puckered lips and filled it in with a lighter lipstick color. We brushed on contour under the cheekbone and across the forehead and every morning glued false eyelashes into place. By the time the 1980s finally came along, a general movement away from that exaggerated styling took place. Hair flowed freely. Farrah Fawcett bangs became a thing of the past. Colors were subtler, although the cruel fashion of needing to look natural, even when you were madeup remained.

A lot has changed since we were little and a lot has remained the same. The days of heavy cold creams are pretty much over. Hairstyles are mostly wash and wear, although many women often mousse, spray and gel to make our hair look thick and natural. Many of us are too busy with careers and families — either having them or trying to create them — to be as absorbed with our faces as we once were. We don't have energy for things that seem to waste precious time anymore. We are also not as gullible as we once were. Yet taking care of ourselves and preserving what elements of youth we can is still essential to our lifestyles. In fact, if there is one constant through all of these decades, it is the desire to have, or seem to have, flawless skin. We bought "natural" products when that was the way to achieve perfection in the '60s and '70s; we bought scientific research when that was the way to take our skin into the '80s; and now the question is: What will we be willing to believe and buy in the '90s?

Those of us in our twenties, thirties, forties and fifties buy a lot of cosmetics. Most product-line development is aimed at us. Cosmetics companies are trying to position their products to meet the primary concerns of the female consumer. What they know about us is that we are growing older and that we are worried about it. They also know that life moves at a frantic pace and we don't have time to waste shopping for makeup and using complicated skin care routines. They know that most of us are concerned about the environment and how pollution, a disappearing ozone layer, and ultra-violet radiation affect our skin. Ecology is another consideration for many women. Issues such as animal testing and recyclable packaging can no longer be glossed over; these have become mainstream topics. And finally, economics will be a major area of concern as women realize that there isn't necessarily a noticeable difference between a $5 lipstick and a $17 lipstick or a $20 skin care routine and a $250 skin care routine.

These considerations are already evident at today's cosmetics counters. The industry is going to take a bit of the natural craze from the '70s and the scientific agenda from the '80s and add an environmental twist for the '90s. This next generation of products won't be as simple-sounding as chamomile astringents or strawberry cleansers, nor will they only rely on their unproven boasts that scientific research has won the battle against wrinkles.

More and more the products of the 1990s will include ingredients that are derived from natural sources, but this time, as I've mentioned, the buzzword to describe them will be "botanical." The products will include sunscreens whenever possible and any other ingredients that can possibly keep the sun and air off the face, whether they do any good or not. Our fear of environmental hazards, be it the sun, pollution, smog, or city air, is what the latest product claims will address. Our limited time will also be a relevant issue, and so don't be surprised if you start seeing more and more labels talking about how fast the products work; no doubt more companies will sell their wares on television so that all you have to do is make a phone call to take care of your beauty needs. To address the trend toward ecological awareness, companies that have stopped testing their products on animals will display that fact proudly on their labels, in their ads and over their counters. Recyclable containers will also promote the glamour industry's "raised-consciousness."

As marketing angles change, competition intensifies, and prices go up, sales techniques will have to improve. The sales forces will become better and better trained. When a consumer resists spending $45 for a moisturizer, the clerk will know better how to handle her objections. The cosmetics counters already demonstrate this modification. Displays are much better organized than ever before, and the sales staff, dressed in their lab coats or company attire, have a good deal of the lingo well practiced. This doesn't mean that what they are saying is accurate, or that they understand what they're saying; it only indicates that the whole cosmetics game, from product marketing to sales development, is getting even more competitive and aggressive.

It's time to do things differently. We are more knowledgeable consumers, we are growing older, and we have a choice. We can choose to buy expensive products in the never-ending hope that they will keep us from looking older, or we can finally recognize that cosmetics on the two ends of the price scale have more in common than they have differences. Many of us have been running in circles around the cosmetics counters for almost three decades now, hoping that each new product we buy will contain the answer for which we've been searching. The sad fact is that we keep stretching our pocket-books to afford what we think is a better product. We don't always get what we paid for.

CHAPTER SIX

Evaluating the Makeup Products of the Major Cosmetics Companies

THE PROCESS

As I went from cosmetics counter to cosmetics counter, to city after city, as my charge card became a bent, bruised blur, I realized that the task I had set out to accomplish was more brutal than I had imagined. The number of products to review was nothing less than overwhelming, the salespeople were everything from patient and polite to rude and insulting, and the total expense was astonishing. To top it off, I was asked to leave several department stores where the staff felt I was conducting inappropriate research at their cosmetics counters. Even writing down names of colors and contents was seen as improper. Through it all, in spite of the hassles, I always felt elated and quite beautiful when the makeup I was testing went on smoothly and the colors looked sensational. I also felt irritated and unattractive when the makeup went on blotchy and the colors looked dreary. My hope is that this research will increase *your* chances of having the former experience and not the latter.

I shopped each cosmetics line thoroughly, evaluating each product for its components, texture, appearance, color, ease of use, application and price. I used basically five criteria: 1) Given what was described on the label, could the product do what it promised? 2) How did the product differ from other products? 3) How intense was the fragrance? 4) Was a moisturizer good, given its ingredients? and 5) How absurd were the products' claims? Keep in mind that developing a preference for texture and for what works well on your own skin comes only from testing products on your own. Chapter Seven will help you learn what to look for in skin care products.

When it came to foundations, I eliminated all orange, pink, green or ashen colors; no one's skin is or should ever be orange, pink, green or ashen. Where I thought a specific color would be good for a particular skin tone, or a specific type of product would be good for a particular kind of skin type, I so indicated. Foundations were also evaluated on consistency, coverage and feel. And, if an oil-free foundation contained ingredients that could cause blemishes, although the label indicated it was non-comedogenic, I noted that as well.

There is an array of products that falls into the category of concealers. These products are supposed to cover blemishes (cover sticks), hide dark circles under the eye (cover sticks, concealers, undereye highlighters), change the color tone of the skin (color primers and tints), and set the eyeshadow on the lid (eyeshadow base or primers). I feel strongly that all but the undereye concealers are a waste of time, money and effort. Use of undereye concealers is an excellent way to make dark circles under the eye look lighter. The problem with many of these concealers, however, is their consistency: They are either too dry, which can make the skin look wrinkly and dehydrated, or they are too greasy, which can cause the makeup to fill in the lines around the eyes. The greasy consistency also promotes smearing of the eyeliner placed along the lower eyelashes. The drier the consistency the less likely the eyeliner will smear, but then your undereye may look dry. Regardless of consistency, many concealers are either too dark, orange, pink or mauve to really lighten dark circles. If the concealer is darker or a radically different color than your foundation tone, it isn't going to work properly. In my book *Blue Eyeshadow Should Be Illegal,* I recommended using a white highlighter that you blend with your foundation to make the undereye look lighter; with white you don't have to worry that the color of the foundation will clash with the color of the concealer. It's still a good idea, but because white undereye concealers can be hard to find, I also recommended very light flesh-tone colors that work with most foundations without turning orange, pink or ashen under the eye.

Finishing powders come in two basic forms: pressed and loose. In my study I found the price variation amongst these products to be another stunning example of how marketing and packaging influence the image and cost of a product. Pressed and loose powders are mostly a combination of talc and mineral oil, or talc and another mineral or starch, and these basic formulations can range in price from $3 to $30. Powders that are talc-free often contain cornstarch or wheatstarch and an assortment of naturally occurring minerals and clays. Talc-based powders are no better than those that are talc-free. If you have oily skin, try to avoid all powders that contain oil. Finishing powders were evaluated on the basis of whether or not they went on chalky, sheer or heavy and with too much pink, peach or rose coloring. I consistently gave higher marks to powders that went on sheer with a natural tan or beige finish.

Although color choice of eyeshadow and blush is a personal one, in my evaluations I did eliminate shades that were too shiny. The main problem with shiny eyeshadows is that they make the skin on the lid look wrinkly and, except for evening wear, they look out of place (the same can be said for shiny blush colors). Texture and ease of application also played a large part in my determination of shadow preference. I was leery of eyeshadow sets that included difficult-to-use color combinations. It goes without saying that I purged shiny bright blues and greens without a second thought.

The hardest products to review were lipsticks. Each woman has her own needs and preferences. Some women like sheerer applications; others require glossy or matte finishes. Color is also difficult to recommend because of the wide variation in taste and wardrobe colors. When it came to appraising lipstick, primarily I reviewed the range of color selection and textures available, citing my personal preferences for creamy lipsticks that went on evenly and weren't glossy or sticky. I overlooked lip glosses unless they were unique in some way, as I usually don't recommend them. Lip glosses don't stay on longer than an hour or two, and most lipsticks nowadays are creamy enough to make the lips feel moist without looking wet and greasy.

Often variations in makeup products are merely reflections of marketing techniques. Nowhere is this more evident than in the category of eye pencils, lip pencils and eyebrow pencils. You'll see some beautiful packaging, and a variety of sizes, colors and, on occasion, textures. Some pencils are greasier or drier than others, but for the most part, pencils have a lot in common. (In fact, if you read the labels, many of them, regardless of the cosmetics line, turn out to be made in Germany.) The eye pencils that smudged and smeared, the lip pencils that were greasy and wouldn't last, and the eyebrow pencils that went on like a crayon were all rated as ineffective. Keep in mind that whether or not an eye pencil smears along the lower eyelashes depends primarily on the type of moisturizer you use around the eye and the type of undereye concealer you use. The greasier the moisturizer or the undereye concealer, the more likely any pencil will smear.

I reviewed mascaras based on their ability to go on easily and quickly while building length and thickness at the same time. I considered brush size and shape only if a brush seemed particularly awkward to use; brush preference is an entirely personal matter. I did not include waterproof mascaras in my review, because I don't recommend them. Waterproof mascara contains a petrolatum-based solvent that is hard on the lashes because it needs to be wiped off (instead of washed off). This process can pull out delicate lashes.

Specialty products such as brushes, eyebrow gels, lipstick sealers, eyelash gels, liquid eyelining pens and two-in-one products (such as a lipstick and lip pencil in one set) were all judged individually, based on their convenience and reliability. Some of these products were remarkable and others, as you can well imagine, were a complete waste of money.

Blush and eyeshadow brushes are carried by some of the major cosmetics lines, and most department stores sell brush sets of some kind. Brush quality was rated on overall shape and function as well as the softness and density of the bristles. An eyeshadow or blush brush that had scratchy, stiff, or loose bristles was not recommended.

As you read my comments, you may find yourself disagreeing with me. That's okay, because the criteria you use to evaluate cosmetics may differ from mine. Or, for any one of a dozen reasons, a product I hate may work well for you. What I present are merely guidelines, my point of view, about what works and what doesn't. If you decide to follow any of my suggestions, be sure to try the specific product if you can before you buy it. None of my recommendations is a guarantee. But at least I may have set you on the path of discovering what does and doesn't work for you.

A few more points about these reviews: Neither the information nor the evaluations are endorsements. Nor do they represent a particular company's sponsorship. Believe me, none of the cosmetics companies paid me for my remarks or time; I think most would prefer to lock me up! They wouldn't even grant me telephone interviews when I inquired about rationales for product formulations.

The following list of brand names is alphabetical, so the order in which they appear does not represent my preference. There is no implied winner among any of the cosmetics companies I included; no one line had all the answers or had a majority of great products. Almost every line had its strong and weak points.

One last comment: I would encourage you to take this book with you on shopping trips to the cosmetics counters or the drugstore. Then you will have all the information you'll need readily at hand. There is no way you can remember the details of each product, color and brand. Do try to be discreet at the department store cosmetics counters — don't be surprised if you find that using the book in clear view of the salespeople makes them defensive or irritated. There are always risks when a consumer comes prepared with information. I urge you to persevere. Nothing will change at the cosmetics counters if you don't change first.

WARNING: All prices and products listed are subject to change. Prices go up and products are discontinued and replaced without notice. Prices of cosmetics sold in drugstores can vary from store to store and they often go on sale. In spite of the erratic pricing of cosmetics, I included price information to give you a basic guideline for comparison. Color suggestions were based either on tester units available at the makeup cosmetics counter, samples (including gifts with a purchase or discounted promotions), and products that were purchased. The color, shade or tone of a particular product can fluctuate for a number of reasons. If I refer to a particular foundation as being "too peach" and you find that it's just right, it may be that we simply disagree or it may be that the tester you used is different from the one I used.

Adrien Arpel

Adrien Arpel is a study in entrepreneurial excellence. Adrien Arpel represents the company she created with finesse and practicality. Regrettably, her finesse doesn't extend to most of her products, which are either too thick and heavy, too out of date or don't work well. For example, all the foundations in her line are supposed to be applied over a mauve "primer" called Porcelain Coverbase, which goes on rather lavender white. That extra layer feels uncomfortable, so for those who like a light makeup application this is not the line to try. Two of the foundation types have colors I don't recommend, and their consistencies are not the best. (Even the salespeople at the Adrien Arpel counters confided that the color choices were poor.) But the Two-In-One Powdery Creme Makeup is quite good and can definitely be used by itself. The eyeshadows in this line are almost all too shiny, which is unfortunate, since you may choose any two or three colors for their duo or trio containers. (The concept is nice because, in theory, you shouldn't end up buying a color you won't use). The blushes are also problematic; they are all rather dull mauve tones, which might be all right for some skin tones, but not if you want a soft, pastel look. Actually the entire color line is, at best, sparse. The lipsticks were good, but the selection was also small.

On the other hand, the service at the Adrien Arpel counters I visited was among the best, with salespeople eager to give you mini-facials (most Arpel counters even have private facial rooms right there in the store) and apply makeup.

Foundation: Adrien Arpel has four types: 1) Sheer Souffle which is for extremely dry skins (it can go on heavy and greasy unless you really know how to blend); 2) Glycerin Liquid which has an unusual slippery texture, gives light to medium coverage, is tricky to blend and might take a bit of getting used to (recommended for oily or combination skin, and most of the colors are for women with darker skin tones); 3) Color Tint Sport Moisturizer is more of a lightweight foundation than it is a tint; and 4) Creme Powder Foundation which has a wonderful consistency and goes on smoothly. (It comes packaged with an undereye concealer, which would be more impressive if the concealer weren't so dark and yellow.)

Foundation Colors to Try

Glycerin Liquid Powder ($20)
> Sable: May be a good color for women of color with dark skin tones.

Creme Powder Foundation ($25)
> All of these are great color choices: Naturelle, Flesh, Nude, Bare and Buff.

Foundation Colors to Avoid

Sheer Souffle ($22)
> All of these colors are either too orange or too pink: Ivory, Fair, Basic and Tan.

Glycerin Liquid Powder ($20)
> All of these colors are too orange: Wheat, Cashmere, Honey and Maple.

Color Tint Sport Moisturizer ($20.50)

All of these colors are too peach: Light, Medium, Dark and Bronzer. (The bronzer is too shiny, but may be ok for darker skin tones for evening wear.)

Concealer: Adrien Arpel has a unique concealer system called Undereye Concealer ($16.50). It is a yellow-orange color too dark for most fair, light and medium skin tones. It is not meant to be worn alone, but blended over a product called Coveraway ($15.50). Coveraway is blue in color and goes on blue. The explanation Arpel gives for this strange color is that blue deflects shadows better than white or light beige. I disagree.

Finishing Powder: Adrien Arpel has three good shades of Pressed Powder ($20). This powder contains lanolin, which can be a problem for women who are allergic to it or have a tendency toward blemishes and blackheads.

Blush: I like Adrien Arpel's concept of offering the consumer an empty container with two sections into which you fit individually packaged tins of blush and contour color. It is a cost-effective idea that prevents you from having to buy a color you won't use in order to get a shade you will. The problem is that selection is limited to darker blush colors. The Powdery Creme Blush also comes in a limited range of colors, but the shades are softer and brighter.

Blush Colors to Try

Mix & Match Cheek Color (two shades plus compact, $19.50;
   refills, $6 per color)
   All of these colors are ok: Contour, Ginger, Apricot, Azalea,
   Natural Pink (more mauve than pink), Pink Mauve and
   Strawberry.
Powdery Creme Blush ($17.50)
   Each of these is a good color choice: Aubergine, Pink, Chocolate
   (good contour color) and Rouge.

Eyeshadow: Much like the blush, having Mix & Match Eyeshadows (two shades plus compact, $19.50; refills, $6 per color) is a great idea, but again the color choice is poor — they're all too shiny. The Powdery Creme Eyeshadow ($14.50) is also hard for me to recommend because I personally find it difficult to use. The colors are also quite shiny, go on dry, are difficult to blend and have a tendency to crease.

Lipstick: Adrien Arpel makes a product called Lipstick Lock ($11.50) that is supposed to prevent lipstick from bleeding into the lines around the mouth and keep the color the same all day. I found that it did not keep the color from shifting and it definitely did not prevent my lipstick from bleeding. There are three types of lipstick in this line: Matte Powder Creme ($15.50) which contains kaolin (clay), goes on rather dry and has a tendency to dry out the lips; Cream Lipstick ($15.50) has a nice consistency but a small selection of colors; Sheer Lipstick ($10.50), which is really a lip gloss in a tube.

Eye, Lip and Brow Pencils: The dual-edge Brow Color ($10) comes in three shades and has a good, dry texture so it won't be shiny on the brow. There are only four shades of Eye Pencil ($10), each with a slick, almost greasy texture that smears. There is also a selection of fat eye pencils called Eye Trimmers ($10). These are difficult to sharpen and can smear during the day. The Lipliners ($16.50) come with one end as a lipstick brush — nice idea and somewhat convenient, but a decent pencil with a separate lipstick brush would be just as effective and less expensive. Adrien Arpel also makes a Brow Gel, but it comes in only one shade and, obviously, that color isn't going to suit everyone.

Mascara: By now it might sound like I'm bashing Adrien Arpel, but I am sorry to say that the mascara ($12.50) smudged and flaked off by the end of a long day.

Specialty Products: Shadow Undercoat ($14.50) for the eyelid, is an unnecessary product because foundation and powder essentially do the same thing. One of the inherent problems with this line, and many other lines, is the ludicrous number of products they want you to use. Case in point: If you use the Shadow Undercoat, the Porcelain Cover-base ($19.50), the Coveraway, Undereye Concealer, *and* foundation, it's quite likely that your face will feel weighed down with makeup.

Almay

Almay has a long-standing reputation as one of the few lines, whether sold at the drugstore or at the cosmetics counters, that is 100 percent hypoallergenic. Given that there are no specific guidelines about what ingredients are less likely to cause allergic reactions, this is an admirable feat. For the most part, Almay does a good job of eliminating well known irritants such as fragrance, formaldehyde compounds, lanolin and lauryl sulfate compounds. But those may not be the ingredients that cause your particular skin problems. Almay has some excellent products worth considering. Though the color selection is a bit sparse, there are several areas in which Almay excels. They make some of the best mascaras, blushes and lipsticks I've tested on the market and they also have a superior undereye concealer that comes in a tube and has a creamy, soft texture.

Foundation: There are no testers available for the Almay foundations. Even the Cream Powder Makeup ($4.95) is packaged in such a way that you can't see the actual color at all, so none of these are being included in this review.

Concealer: Almay's Cover-Up Stick ($3.50) is a superior concealer that comes in three workable shades: Light, Medium and Dark. The lipstick-like applicator helps it to go on creamy, but not greasy, and it tends not to crease in the lines around the eye. This one is definitely worth looking into, although the consistency may be too moist for oily-skin types. There is also an Undereye Cover Cream ($3.50) that comes in a pot in three excellent shades: Light, Medium and Dark. It is somewhat greasy, although it is good for dry skin and doesn't crease in the lines around the eye; Almay's Waterproof Extra Protection Concealer ($4.05) also comes in three shades; Ivory, Light and Medium. Although I like the shades, I don't recommend using a waterproof anything.

Finishing Powder: Almay has two types of pressed powder; Shine Free Blotting Powder ($4.65) and Sheer Finish ($4.65). They are almost identical; both are talc-based, although the Shine Free does not contain mineral oil. Both of these are very good. The colors are neutral without peach or pink overtones. Definitely an inexpensive, but reliable powder to consider.

Blush: Almay has a small, but excellent selection of blushes. There is little difference between the Cheek Color blush and the Brush-On Blush except that the latter has an attractive mirror compact. The Cream Powder blush is outstanding and the colors go on very soft.

Blush Colors to Try
Cheek Color ($3.95)
> All these colors are beautiful: Mauve, Rose, Soft Pink, Peach, Fusccchia, Plum, Cherry, Mid Pink, Apricot, Blush and Soft Bronze (good contour color).

Brush-On Blush ($6.50)
> All these colors are beautiful: Tawny Rose, Dune Blossom, Sunlit Peach, Hint of Mauve, Pure Pinkberry, Soft Apricot, Damask Rose and Silkberry.

Cream Powder Blush ($6.50)
> All these colors are great: Rosewood, Crystal Mauve, Pink Sand and Primrose.

Blush Colors to Avoid
Brush-On Blush ($6.50)
> Shimmering Pink.

Eyeshadow: For the most part, Almay does not have the best eyeshadows I've seen on the market. The colors are too shiny and the selection extremely limited. Their 8-Hour eyeshadow colors I tried lasted longer than eight hours, yet I wonder why Almay markets an eyeshadow that lasts less time than most women would consider reasonable. Their Waterproof Eyeshadow Pencil ($4) comes in colors that are too shiny to recommend or colors that are difficult to use — tones such as Marine Blue, Yellow and Bright Teal. The waterproofing is also a problem because of the difficulty in removing it when you cleanse your face.

Eyeshadow Colors to Try
Singles ($2)
> Fawn: Good color choice.
> African Violet: Good color choice.

Eyeshadow Colors to Avoid
8-Hour Color ($4.95)
> All of these colors are extremely shiny: Crystal Violet, Sunset, Night Sky, Moonrose, Thunderstorm, Tradewind.

Singles ($2)
> All of these colors are extremely shiny: Topaz, Tapestry, Platinum,

Pebble Beach, Rose Fresco, Island Breeze, Champagne, Organdy, Sherbet and Batik (too blue).

Lipstick: Almay has a small but attractive selction of lip colors ($4.65) that go on soft and perfectly creamy.

Lip, Eye and Brow Pencil: Almay has an excellent, albeit small, selection of automatic Lipcolor Pencils ($3.95) with a dry, but smooth, texture. There are several eyelining products: All Day Shadow Liner ($4.50) comes in colors that are too bright to recommend; Kohl-Formula Eye Pencil ($4.75) has a sponge-tip at one end and, in spite of the limited color selection, is a good basic pencil; Skip Proof Eye-lining Pen ($4.95) is a felt-tip liquid liner that comes in navy, black and brown. The Kohl-Formula Eye Pencil is very good, but not exceptional, just like most of the pencils on the market.

Mascara: Almay makes some of the best mascaras on the market. Both One Coat Mascara ($2) and Mascara Plus ($2.50) create beautiful lashes without clumping or smearing, and the price is right!

Specialty Products: Touch on Blemish Treatment ($4.95) is nothing more than foundation that contains sulfur in a tube. Sulfur won't heal an acne lesion and it can be irritating to the skin.

The Body Shop

I wish I could say only wonderful things about The Body Shop, because there are many things about this extremely successful corporation that I respect and admire. An English-based company specializing in natural-sounding inexpensive shampoos, cleansers and bath products, The Body Shop is an entrepreneur's dream come true. Starting with only one small storefront in London, it has grown to hundreds of shops all over America, Europe and Australia. Besides the impressive growth, The Body Shop has taken the tradition of beauty and skin care and turned it into a political, philosophical venture . Their basic credo is that looking good is important but not at the cost of hurting animals. None of their products is tested on animals. The in-store literature and window displays tell more about these issues than about skin or hair care. I admire the humane philosophy mixed with good old-fashioned capitalism. It's nice to be reminded that you can earn a living and still stand by your beliefs.

Having said all that, I regret to say that I don't care for their products very much. Most of the skin care items contain ingredients that are nothing special. Several contain preservatives that are irritating, and their makeup products are best described as mediocre. The small cosmetics display area in the stores is quite accessible and you are free to play with the demos all you want. This lack of pressure is the consequence of hiring store personnel who are not trained to be makeup or skin care experts. There are no sales speeches, but there is also no "expertise" to be found here. If you know what you're looking for, it's a wonderful way to shop. The products sell themselves and the prices are reasonable to downright inexpensive. (By the way, even though I don't care for their skin care products, they do come in small trial sizes so that if you disagree with me, or want to explore on your own, you can try them for a minimal amount of money.)

Foundation: The Body Shop has two types of foundation: All-in-One-Face Base ($14.95) that goes on either dry or wet and is extremely sheer, although it can look somewhat powdery; and Liquid Foundation ($5.45) that goes on light in a silky smooth texture. The problem with both of these foundations isn't quality, but the limited number of colors. The foundation coverage is light and the products blend easily enough, although they are not for everyone. The nice colors which are available merit a try. The price of their Liquid Foundation in particular is definitely worth the cost.

Concealer: Of all their makeup products, the Concealers ($3.75) are the best. They go on smooth, with a slightly drier texture than most, which is great for oily-skin types, and the color choices are great. I would not recommend this one for dry skin.

Finishing Powder: There are two Pressed Powder ($8.75) colors. Both are ok but may go on chalky.

Blush: The blushes at The Body Shop, both cream and powder ($4.75), are definite possibilities, but the color choices are limited: 01 is a bit shiny, 02 is good, 03 and 04 are great.

Eyeshadow: A small, shiny color selection makes these eyeshadows ($4.50) hard to recommend except for two: 02 is a nice rose-peach color and 06 is a soft plum. The Eyeshadow Pencils ($6.50) look more convenient to use than they are. The color glides on easily, but the tips are difficult to keep sharpened. They are also too shiny to recommend.

Lipstick: The Body Shop has a small selection of lip glosses called Liptints ($4.85). They stain the lips with a slight color which remains once the gloss part wears off. They are too greasy-looking for me to recommend for a daytime business look, but they can be acceptable, if you blot after you apply the Liptint.

Eye and Lip Pencils: All the eye pencils ($3.75) are good, usable colors except for the vivid blue and green ones. The lip pencils ($3.75) are also good, basic colors with a nice, smooth texture.

Brushes: These are some of the nicest brushes (priced $2.95 to $5.95) on the market. The blush brush is soft and a perfect size, as are the eyeshadow brushes. The only brush I don't recommend is the lip brush or foam applicator stick.

Borghese

I have to admit that Borghese stands out, if for no other reason than its singularly Italian flavor in the midst of so many French and American lines. It is also one of the more expensive manufacturers. Regardless of the price tag, the products I liked, I really liked, and the ones I disliked, I really disliked. For example, Borghese has some of the most velvety smooth foundations, particularly their new foundations — Milano 2000 (there are often samples available of this one), Lumina Compact Foundation, and Liquid Powder Foundation — although they tend to be too fragrant. Their new blush, Liquid Powder Blush, is also quite remarkable. The eyeshadows, on the other hand, are beautiful to look at in the container but are too shiny to recommend, as are the regular blushes, although they do go on smoothly. Be careful with all of the Borghese products; many of them are overly fragranced.

Borghese has very accessible counter displays that are organized loosely into three color groupings: Oro (yellow-based), Rosso (pink-based) and Neutrale (neutral/beige). These groupings are helpful but a bit more confusing than some of the other cosmetic lines that divide their colors into the traditional four color families. The salespeople I encountered, albeit fairly aggressive, were well trained. They seemed to know their sales manual backward and forward.

Foundation: Borghese has three foundation types that are all excellent: Milano 2000 is a liquid foundation that goes on smooth and velvety and works well for dry skin, although it does have a strong fragrance. Liquid Powder makeup is unique and works well on somewhat flawless, normal skin. If you have any dry skin at all, you may find this foundation, which goes on wet and dries to a powder, looks tight and flaky. Lumina Compact Foundation is quite light, although it looks as if it would go on heavy and thick. This is a nice, convenient way to put on foundation and would work well for women who want a matte moist look to their makeup and have normal skin. All three are worth a try, in spite of the ultra-steep price tag.

Foundation Colors to Try

Milano 2000 ($45)
Rosso 1: Good color although it may turn pink on some skin tones.

Rosso 4: For dark skin tones only; may turn orange.

Rosso 5: For dark skin tones only; may turn slightly orange.

Oro 1: Perfect color for fair skin tones.

Oro 2: Perfect color for fair skin tones.

Oro 3: Okay color for darker skin tones, although it may turn orange.

Oro 4: Great color for darker skin tones.

Oro 5: Great color for darker skin tones.

Neutrale 1: Perfect color for fair skin tones.

Neutrale 2: Perfect color for fair skin tones.

Neutrale 3: Perfect color for medium skin tones.

Neutrale 4: Ok color for medium to dark skin tones, although it may turn pink or rose.

Neutrale 5: Ok color for darker skin tones, although it may turn orange.

Liquid Powder Makeup ($35)
All shades are excellent.

Lumina Compact Foundation ($42.50)
All colors are excellent, but still are slightly shiny: Peretta Beige,

Peretta Fresco, Soft Bronzed, Solari Beige, Alabastro, Ivory Lustro, Beige D'Oro and Golden Biscotti (which may be too ashy for most skin tones).

Foundation Colors to Avoid

Milano 2000 ($45)
Rosso 2: Too pink for anyone's skin tone.
Rosso 3: Again, too pink for anyone's skin tone.
Liquid Powder Makeup ($35)
Rosso 1: Too orange.
Rosso 2: Too orange.
Neutrale 4: May be too ashy for many skin tones.

Concealer: Borghese has a two-in-one product called Eye Makeup Primer ($17) that comes in a tube; one end is for the lid and the other is the concealer for under the eye or over blemishes. Both colors are good and have a decent texture, although I think that a lid primer is an unnecessary step. The undereye concealer is ok, but if you only use that and not the primer you aren't getting much product for the $17 price tag.

Finishing Powder: Borghese has a titanium dioxide (opaque white mineral) and talc-based pressed powder ($27.50) that goes on very soft and comes in excellent colors: Rosso, Neutrale 1, Neutrale 2 and Neutrale 3 are all nice; Oro may look a bit peach on some skin tones. The loose powder ($27.50) also contains titanium dioxide and talc.

Blush: Borghese makes a unique blush called Liquid Powder Blush. This new way of applying blush is relatively easy to use. It sounds trickier than it is, although application can take a bit of getting used to. It doesn't work well over dry skin and is best suited for normal or oily skin. The Liquid Powder Blush goes on wet, dries to a powder with a rather smooth matte appearance, and the color stays on well. The product comes packaged with a brush and small sponge; the sponge is probably easier to use, but it all depends on your preference. All the colors are worth a try, particularly if you are looking for something different in a blusher. Unfortunately, most of the colors are all slightly shiny, but not shiny enough to make a difference; it is still an excellent product to consider. The regular blush colors are also all quite lovely, and the texture soft and satiny.

Blush Colors to Try

Liquid Powder Blush ($30)

Milano Tulle: Good color, but somewhat shiny.

Milano Rossore: Good color to try.

Milano Vino: Good color for dark skin tones.

Milano Terrecotte: Too shiny; for evening wear only.

Regular Blush ($27)

Pelates: Very shiny red, but can be a good evening blush color for darker skin tones.

Coralino: Lovely soft coral.

Rose Brillante: Great rose color.

Rosetto: Beautiful color.

Pesca: Beautiful color.

Abbronzato: Too shiny, but can be a good evening blush color.

Peach Biscotti: Excellent contour color.

Frascati: Excellent contour color for fair skin tones.

Coral Eletrico: Can be too orange for most skin tones.

Plumage: Slightly shiny, strong pink shade.

Ametista: A unique, somewhat lavender shade of blush.

Pink Marabue: Slightly shiny.

Peonia: Great soft pink.

Coral Aida: Beautiful color.

Garnet Boheme: Beautiful color.

Natural Finish Bronzer: Good contour color, but do not use alone.

Eyeshadow: Borghese makes an appealing assortment of eyeshadow colors that have inconsistent texture and almost all have too much shine. Some have a great silky texture and go on soft, while others feel very heavy and go on quite thick. The shadows called Quartetto are foursomes of color arranged in a mosaic-like pattern, which looks pretty but is actually difficult to use with a decent-sized eyeshadow brush.

Eyeshadow Colors to Try

Singles, Duos, Trios and Quads ($22 – $30)

Grafite: Great slate gray.

Avorio: Nice pale pink, but may be too white for most skin tones.

Quarzo: Lovely soft pink.

Rocco: Great brown shade for lining and shading.

Romanza: Bright but interesting matte combination of pale yellow, pale peach and pale lime green.
Aida: Beautiful and soft combination.
La Boheme: A beautiful trio of colors.
Madame Butterfly: Beautiful soft combination.

Eyeshadow Colors to Avoid

Singles, Duos, Trios and Quads ($22 – $30)

All of these colors are too shiny: Azurite (intensely blue), Botania, Siena, Amore, Geocolorie, Sculture, Rubio and Ametista (may be good for evening wear on darker skin tones), Moderno (not shiny, but difficult combination) and Opalinos (evening wear only).

Lipstick: Borghese sells three types of lipstick in a limited selection of color. One has a moisturizing center. Lip Treatment Moisturizer ($17), is very greasy and is more like a lip gloss than a lipstick. Another is a set of shiny lipsticks that go on rather dry and iridescent. The third is a matte lipstick called La Moda Concentrate ($17) that goes on matte and rather dry. La Moda wears well, yet although the claim on the package says it won't feather (bleed into the lines around the mouth), it did for me. It didn't feather as much as some lipsticks I've worn, but it definitely did bleed some, plus the dry texture isn't the most comfortable on the lips. They also have a new set of powder lip colors called Lip Colour Superlativo. Even if I liked the concept of powdered lip colors, and I don't, all of these shades are intensely shiny and make the mouth look rather wrinkled.

Eye, Brow and Lip Pencils: The eye pencils ($17) are simply basic pencils in a good array of colors that are mostly shiny; one end has a sponge tip to blend the color. Borghese also has a very good brow gel in limited colors called Brow Milano ($17). Unfortunately, there are no shades for ash, dark brown or black brow color. The lip pencils ($17) come in a good array of colors but are slightly on the greasy side.

Mascara: Borghese's Volumina Luxuriant Mascara ($16) has a wand unlike most others on the market. One side is smooth with grooves, and the other has small stiff bristles. I didn't care for this product at all: I found it hard to use, it did not lengthen my lashes and it flaked and smeared as the day went by.

Chanel

The people at Chanel counters across the country really have their acts together. I guess when your cosmetics are this expensive, you have no other choice. The salespeople dress in a Chanel uniform and are very enthusiastic about the fact that Chanel has its origins in France, never mind that none of the products seems to be manufactured there. For the most part, I did not find Chanel to be an exceptional product line. None of the Chanel products impressed me as being worth the expense. The foundations were ok and the mascara was good, but not great; the lipsticks were quite good and the way they were arranged by color was very helpful, but, again, I'm not convinced they're worth the steep price. A handful of their products also contain 2-Bromo-2 Nitropane-1, 3 Diol, a preservative that is considered to cause dermatitis. Chanel is definitely a prestige line, and most of the women I interviewed believed that they got something special for their money, though no one was exactly sure what that something special was.

Chanel's counter displays are set up in such a way that you need a salesperson to help you test the products. All of their blushes, lipsticks, eye and lip pencils are attractively divided into very helpful color groupings called Les Violettes (pink/plum), Les Rose Bleus (red/blue), Les Naturels (soft tones of brown/peach) and Les Soleils (yellow/coral). These are then subdivided by intensity. The eyeshadows are grouped similarly, but I was confused about how some of the shades relate to their color groups. Some Chanel counters have a device that asks you questions about your hair and eye color; this is to help place you within a set range of foundation choices. When I tried it, the foundation suggestion was much too dark for my skin tone.

Based on their color groupings and intensity categories, Chanel claims that any woman can wear any color group (yellow tones, blue tones, pink tones and natural tones, according to their charts) as long as she wears the correct intensity of the color. That may be a valid theory, but most women who know their colors would disagree. If you are interested in trying a different color palette, you may be curious enough to give this a try, but be very skeptical. I think that it's just another angle to sell more products.

Chanel eyeshadows tend to be too shiny and too intense — they don't produce what I would call a subtle look at all. The consistency of their eyeshadows and blushes, however, is sensational. The eyeshadows have the new quilted texture that is supposed to prevent cracking and flaking. Many companies use this new pressing pattern, but it makes no difference in their products' duration or strength. At almost $50 each, I find Chanel eyeshadows too expensive to even look at.

Foundation: Chanel's foundations are good, but they too are expensive and come in an extremely limited color selection. They are in the process of discontinuing one of their foundations designed for oily skins called Teint Pur because it contained iridescence (how many women with oily skin want a foundation that shines?); their new oil-free foundation Teint Pur Matte no longer has the shine, but it does contain aluminum starch which can be a skin irritant. The other foundations Teint Naturel and Teint Creme for dry skin are a better bet, although I definitely prefer the colors and texture of the Teint Naturel. However, all these foundations contain much too much fragrance for my taste.

Chanel has an under makeup base called Perfect Colour Matte, Perfect Colour Creme and Perfect Colour Pearle ($50 each). These semi-opaque tints lay a sheer white layer over the face, supposedly to make the skin look fair and flawless. It's hard for me to understand this one. In my opinion these undercoats make the skin look chalky. The Pearle is being discontinued — the shine was almost impossible to get off the face and it did strange things to the foundation. Perfect Colour Bronze and Perfect Colour Blush ($50 each) are two of the sheerest face tints you'll find on the market — best for fair to medium skin tones only. All these products contain a SPF of 8 which is nice, but not enough to protect the face from the sun.

Foundation Colors to Try

Teint Pur Matte ($37)
   All of these colors are great: Ivory, Soft Bisque, Natural Beige. Golden Beige (good color but can turn orange on some skin tones).

Teint Naturel ($47.50)
   All these colors are great: Natural Beige, Golden Beige, Tawny Beige, Soft Bisque, Alabaster and Porcelain.

Teint Creme ($47.50)
   All of these colors are great: Tawny Beige, Golden Beige, Soft Bisque, Alabaster and Pale Ivory.

Foundation Colors to Avoid

Teint Pur Matte ($37)
> Alabaster: May be too pink for most skin tones.
> Tawny Beige: May be too orange for some skin tones.

Teint Creme ($47.50)
> Natural Beige: May be too peach for most skin tones.
> Pale Ivory: Too pink for most skin tones.

Concealer: Chanel's undereye Cover Sticks ($20) have a slightly greasy texture and the colors are not the best. The Professional shade is too blue and combines poorly with the foundation. The Light shade is slightly pink, but may be acceptable for some skin tones. The medium shade can turn slightly rosy. These won't crease and the stick applicator is convenient, but there are better and cheaper ones on the market.

Finishing Powder: Chanel's Loose Powder ($30) and Luxury Pressed Powder ($42.50) tend to go on very chalky in spite of their lovely silky texture. Medium is the best shade, and works for fair-skinned women only. The Bronze shade, designed for women of color, is too orange for most darker skin tones. The colors Mauve, Pink, Peach, Pink Champagne appear too chalky on the skin to recommend.

Blush: For the most part Chanel's blush colors have a splendid silky texture, but some are too intense for most skin types and most are too shiny. Their blushes also contain cornstarch, an ingredient that can clog pores.

Blush Colors to Try

All Blush Colors ($27.50)
> Rose Quartz 2: Good pink-peach shade but somewhat shiny.
> Peach Flame: Very bright orange; more for dark skins only, but
>   be careful.
> Mauve 3: Good color but somewhat shiny.
> Cherry 2: Very pretty color though somewhat shiny.
> Peach Salon: This shade of peach is too orange for most skin
>   tones, but this one isn't shiny.
> Tempting Beige: Interesting shade of mauve with a hint of peach,
>   somewhat shiny.
> Fuschia 1: Good color.
> Red Fire: For dark complexions only.

Blush Colors to Avoid

Peony: Very bright pink and very shiny.
Pink Satin 2: A soft color but very shiny.
Natural Pink: Fairly shiny but a beautiful color.
Rose Quartz: Fairly shiny but a beautiful color.

Eyeshadow Colors to Try

All Eyeshadow Colors ($47.50)
Black: Good color.
Les Mats Naturels 4: Great colors to try.
Les Mats 5: Great colors to try.

Eyeshadow Colors to Avoid

All the following colors are too shiny: Champagne/Midnight,
Charcoal/Opal, Tumultes, Les Coromandel, Les Tropiques, Les
Pastels, Les Tentations, Nuances, Les Ocres, Forest/Sunset, Sand/
Seagreen, Peach/Sable, Violet/Turquoise, Gold/Silver, Shadow,
Champagne, Mist Smoke, Yellow, Peach, Chamois, Taupe, Navy,
Amethyst, and Purple Smoke, Escabrilles (is slightly shiny) and
Emerald (is too green and slightly shiny).

Lipstick: Chanel makes one of the few lip products that works to keep
lipstick from bleeding into the lines around the mouth; it is called
Protective Colour Control ($18.50). Unfortunately, one of the side
effects of using this product is its tendency to become caked on the lips
as you apply more lipstick over it, and it's expensive. The price may be
worth it for those who suffer from feathering, but I did find cheaper
drug store products which worked as well. I also liked Chanel's Rouge a
Levres ($17) very much. The texture is somewhat creamy and matte, not
greasy feeling as are many of the lipsticks you find on the market today.

Lip, Brow and Eye Pencils: Chanel's Crayon Contour Des Levres
($21.50) for the lips resembles a dozen other lip pencils on the market
except that it has a lip brush on one end. It is convenient, but it doesn't
warrant the steep price tag! The same holds true for Chanel's eye and
brow pencils, called Smudge Eyeliner ($21.50): one end is a sponge tip
for blending. Be careful, many of these pencil colors are iridescent.

Mascara: Chanel's Luxury Creme Mascara ($17.50) is a good mascara
that goes on easily, doesn't smudge, and builds thick lashes.

Charles of the Ritz

Charles of the Ritz seems to be one of the lesser known department store cosmetics lines. It is considered to be a low-to-medium-priced line, and for the most part that's true. There is an impressive range of products to consider, but the line is a mixed bag of terrific, mediocre and poor ones. The display unit is a bit confusing, but the basic concept is a good one. The board is divided into four palette groups; Red Light Palette, Red Dark Palette, Golden Light Palette and Golden Dark Palette. Only the eyeshadows and blushes are divided into these color group-ings, and the color choices for each group are ok but not great. It would be helpful if the lipsticks, powders and pencils were also divided accordingly. The salespeople for the most part were friendly but not aggressive, making Charles of the Ritz a very approachable makeup line.

Foundation: Charles of the Ritz makes five different foundations that are really quite good: Superior Moisture Foundation (for normal to dry skin) provides medium coverage; Superior Foundation (for normal to oily skin) goes on light and feels great; Perfect Finish has a smooth finish and wonderful color selection but contains alcohol and smells some-what medicinal; Revenescence (for dry skin) has a silky texture but poor color selection; and Powderful Foundation, which is more like a pressed powder than a foundation. I recommend using Powderful Foundation as a pressed powder only; the color selection is excellent, but when used by itself, the skin may look dull and powdery.

Foundation Colors to Try

Perfect Finish ($10)

Milkwood: Great color choice.

Oh So Bare: Good color choice, may turn slightly pink.

The Naked Truth: Good color choice, may turn slightly pink.

Sugar Baby Blush: Excellent neutral beige tone.

Sunny Disposia: Excellent color choice.

Honey Do: Excellent color choice for medium skin tones.

Sandpiper: Great tan shade.

Tisket-a-Bisquit: Ok tan shade, but can turn rose.

My Sinnamon: Excellent color for medium skin tones.

Superior Moisture ($17.50)

Natural Ivory: Good color for extremely fair skin tones, can turn slightly pink.

Soft Beige: Great neutral color for fair to medium skin tones.
New Beige: Good color for medium skin tones, but can turn pink.
Bronzed Beige: Great tan shade.
Superior ($17.50)
Sunlit Beige: Good color for fair skin tones, but may turn pink.
Simply Beige: Great neutral shade for fair skin tones.
Toffee Beige: Nice tan color, but may turn slightly peach.
Warmed-Up Beige: Good medium shade, but can turn pink.
Toasted Beige: Great medium shade.
Revenescence ($25)
Ivory Beige: Great color for medium skin tones.
Sienna Beige: Great bronze color for darker skin tones.
Warm Beige: Good color for medium skin tones, but can turn
    slightly pink.

Foundation Colors to Avoid

Superior Moisture ($17.50)
Beige Sand: Can be too rose for most skin tones.
Deep Beige: Can be a good medium skin tone, but may turn rose.
Beige Blush: Can be a good medium skin tone, but may turn rose.
Tender Beige: Can be too peach for most skin tones.
Superior ($17.50)
Beige Sand: Can be a good color for medium skin tones, but may
    turn peach.
Real Tawny Beige: Can be a good color for medium skin tones,
    but may turn peachy pink.
Peach Beige: Too peach for most skin tones.
Revenescence ($25)
Tawny Beige: Too peach for most skin tones.
Sand Beige: Too peach for most skin tones.
Bronzed Beige: Too rose for most skin tones.
Honey Beige: Too pink for most skin tones.

Concealer: Charles of the Ritz makes a liquid concealer in a tube
called Perfect Instant Concealer ($11). It comes in two colors: Light and
Medium. The light is too pink for most fair or medium skin tones, and
the medium is good only for darker skin tones. The consistency is
slightly dry, but can be acceptable for oily skin types.

Finishing Powder: Charles of the Ritz has an excellent selection of powders called Ready Blended Pressed Powders ($20). The colors are all soft and the texture smooth.

Finishing Powder Colors to Try
Ready Blended Pressed Powders ($13.50)

Perfect Beige: Great color for fair to medium skin tones.
Rose Beige: Good color for medium skin tones.
Bronzed Beige: Great color for medium to dark skin tones.
Pink Sand: Good color for fair skin tones, no pink here.
Classic Ivory: Great color for fair skin tones.

Finishing Powder Colors to Avoid
Ready Blended Bronzers ($20)

All these colors are too shiny: Rose Bronze, Sun Bronze, Copper Bronze, and Gold Bronze.

Blush: Charles of the Ritz has a beautiful assortment of blush colors ($12.50) with a silky, sheer texture. Even the vivid colors can go on soft. All the colors are nice to work with: Gingerly, Simply Peach, Teddy Bare, Funny Valentine, Rosalie, My Little Pinky and Mauve-by-Jove.

Eyeshadow Colors to Try *(excellent selection of matte shades)*
Singles and Trios ($10/$15)

Rapunzel: Interesting shade of yellow.
Brown Bag: Great soft tan shade.
Sassy Little Rose: Great soft, plum-brown shade.
Sand Box: Excellent neutral pale tan color.
Tell-Tale Heart: Great plum shade for darker skin tones.
Lovey Dovey: Excellent shade of soft gray.
Thyme Out: Soft shade of khaki green, can be good accent color for some skin tones.
Champagne & Rose: Great color combination.
Cafe Society: Good color combination for darker skin tones.
Playing with Fire: Good color combination for fair skin tones.
Chasing Rainbows: Good color combination, although the pink shade is somewhat shiny.
Hazy & Blue: Good color combination, except for the blue shade.
Suite Dream: Good color combination, except the tan shade is too shiny.

Swan Song: Good color combination, except the silver-gray shade is too shiny.

Eyeshadow Colors to Avoid
Singles and Trios ($10/$15)
Pennywise: Too shiny.
Angel Eyes: Difficult color combination for most skin tones.
Sweet & Glow: Difficult color combination for most skin tones.
Emerald City: Difficult color combination for most skin tones.

Lipstick: Charles of the Ritz has two types of lipstick to choose from. One is called Powderful Lipstick ($8), the other, Moisture Wear Lipstick ($10), which has a good, creamy consistency in a nice selection of colors. The Powderful lipstick contains — as the name indicates — powder and goes on matte and somewhat dry. After a week or two you may find that your lips are getting chapped and dried out. You would be better off using a creamy lipstick with a lip sealer underneath that prevents lipstick from feathering into the lines around the mouth.

Eye, Brow and Lip Liners: Charles of the Ritz is one of the few lines that makes an eyebrow gel called Brow Definer ($8) in various shades to match the existing brow color. The colors are Doe, Blonde, Foxy, Steel and Crystal (no color). The product is excellent and the brush easy to use. The bristles are long enough to prevent the brow from getting clumpy or thick, as can happen with some of the other gels on the market. The only negative thing is the lack of color choice for women with darker-colored eyebrows. The darkest shade is Doe and that's really a light brown color. All of the lip pencils ($10) come in a somewhat greasy texture that can smear. The eye pencils ($10) have a drier texture and tend to last the whole day.

Mascara: Charles of the Ritz mascara is called Perfect Finish ($9). It is an average mascara that can definitely smudge by the end of the day.

Christian Dior

Dior is a great name when it comes to fashion, but it has lost its footing in the world of makeup. There is nothing particularly outstanding in this line. The eyeshadows are all extremely shiny and the color combinations somewhat difficult. It is one of the few lines with a five-color eyeshadow set, but the colors are almost all too shiny to recommend other than for evening wear. The foundations come in a very limited selection of colors and although I like some of the textures and coverage very much, the manufacturer charges a fairly hefty sum for makeup that is not particularly special or unique. In spite of the limited foundation choices, the pressed powders come in eight different shades, of which only a few are really worth trying. The lipsticks are fairly creamy, but the fragrance can be a bit overwhelming. The counter displays are nice enough and easily accessible, but the colors aren't organized by color families, which can make finding your color range difficult.

Foundation: Christian Dior has four types of foundation, each of which has wonderful smooth silky textures but limited color choices. All of them contain oil, which means there isn't one to recommend for oily skin. Teint d'Ete is a very light, sheer foundation that comes in a pump container; Teint Dior is a light foundation designed for normal to dry skin; Teint Actuel is a thicker, creamier foundation for extremely dry skin that blends better than you would think from the look of it; and Teint Poudre is a pressed powder that is talc-and-oil-based. This powder is slightly heavier than most and it is to be used either as an all-over foundation or as a powder. I recommend the latter; when used as a foundation, I think a powder like this can look pasty.

Foundation Colors to Try

Teint d'Ete ($35)
> Claire d'Ete: Great color.
> Blond d'Ete: Great color.
> Or d'Ete: Great color.

Teint Dior ($35)
> Moyen Rose: Good neutral tan color, but may turn orange on some skin tones.
> Presque Beige: Good neutral beige tone.

Teint Actuel ($35)
> Beige Delicat: Great color.
> Beige Dore: Great medium to tan color.
> True Beige: Good medium to tan color, but can turn peachy-yellow.

Teint Poudre ($25)
> Champagne: Good neutral beige tone.
> Spice: Good tan shade.

Dune: Good neutral beige tone.

Seigle: Good neutral tone.

Opaline: Good shade for fair skin tones.

Foundation Colors to Avoid

Teint d'Ete ($35)

Terre d'Ete: Too orange for most skin tones.

Matin d'Ete: Too orange for most skin tones.

Teint Dior ($35)

Moyen Beige: May turn orange on some skin tones.

Claire Beige: May turn pink on some skin tones.

Tres Claire Beige: Too pink.

Teint Actuel ($35)

Rose Tendre: Too pink for most skin tones.

Rose Beige: Too peach for most skin tones.

Teint Poudre ($25)

Melon: Can be too peach for most skin tones.

Concealer: Christian Dior has a concealer called Precise Cream Corrector ($16) that comes in a tube and has a fairly dry, thick consistency. One shade is fairly pink and the other a peach tone. Both are presently being discontinued and being replaced with a stick-type concealer, that wasn't available for review at the time this book went to press.

Finishing Powder: There are eight pressed powder shades ($27) to choose from, though several are strange colors I would not recommend: Tender Green (why green?), Pale Mauve, White Porcelain (goes on too white), Florentine Blonde (too orange for most skin tones) and Scandinavian Rose (too pink for all skin tones). The three pressed powders that come in natural skin shades are good; they have a soft consistency and go on sheer — Invisible Plus (has a slight pink tint), Sahara Beige and Summer Sun (great color for tan skin tones).

Blush Colors to Try

Blush Final ($28)

All of these blushes have a wonderful silky consistency and texture: Accent (slightly shiny), Soft (great color), Delicat (great color), Attractive (great color), Contour (excellent contour color), and Subtle (too shiny for daytime wear).

Eyeshadow Colors to Try
Duos and Quints ($26/$46)

Siam: Great combination for evening wear, only for dark skin tones.

Scintillating: Great combination for evening wear, but extremely shiny.

Discretion: Great combination; the tan and peach shades are matte and the auburn brown shades are slightly shiny. ·

Pearl: For evening wear only, interesting assortment of opalescent.

Pansies: Great combination for evening wear, but very shiny.

Mist: Beautiful combination and *no shine!*

Monochrome: Difficult combination and very shiny, but worth considering for a unique evening look.

Eyeshadow Colors to Avoid
Duo & Quint Sets ($26/$46)

All of these eyeshadow colors are too shiny to recommend: Bouquets, Extreme Blue, Surprise, Images, Caviar/Vodka, Frost/ Violet, Terre/Earth, Gold/Brown, Forest/Dune, Havana/Rose, Dawn/Dusk, Champagne/Blue, Ocean/ Mauve, Praline/ Liquorice, Cafe/Creme, Champagne/Blue Champagne.

Lipstick: Dior's lipsticks ($16) are all fairly creamy and some colors have a light, matte appearance, but the intense fragrance makes them hard to recommend.

Brow Pencil: There are three shades of brow pencil ($16). Each has a rather dry texture and a brush at one end. Even though I don't care to use a pencil on a brow, this one isn't bad, although any pencil with a similar texture and a separate brow brush could function as well.

Mascara: Christian Dior has an excellent mascara ($15) that goes on quickly and lengthens the lashes quite nicely, but I found much less expensive mascaras on the market that can do the same thing.

Clinique

If the space a cosmetics company takes up at a department store indicates how well the line is doing, then Clinique is doing quite well — their counter space usually takes up the most area. This line seems to be associated more with the young consumer. The products, particularly those for skin care, are aimed at oily- or combination-skin types, which is probably why Clinique attracts a young clientele. And the makeup line includes products and colors that are geared toward younger tastes, with items such as color rubs and tints for the cheek, very sheer blushes and eyeshadows, and a clever variety of eye pencils. Unfortunately, almost all of the pencils, eyeshadows and color rubs are extremely shiny and not the best for daytime.

Many women, regardless of age, are faithful Clinique customers, some because they believe that the products are hypoallergenic and better for their skin; which they aren't. The salespeople, dressed in their white lab coats, reinforce this belief. There are several counter displays available, but most of the products can be tested only with the help of a salesperson. The line has no color philosophy; the color products are not arranged by skin tone, which leaves you at the mercy of the salespeople. In spite of my hesitation about the counter organization, I am impressed with Clinique's large selection of foundations, lipsticks and blushes, all of which are quality products that tend to go on softer and sheerer than most. The price range of the products is also more comfortable than at other counters.

Foundation: Clinique has seven foundations designed for different skin types; I've reviewed six of them. Their Stay True Oil-Free is one of the best oil-free foundations on the market and the color choices are great. The Balanced Makeup Base, for normal to dry skin, is also quite good and the colors are excellent. Extra Help makeup has a nice consistency and would be good for extremely dry skin, except that most of the colors are too pink or peach. The only foundation I don't recommend is the Pore Minimizer. It contains alcohol which is irritating, it provides little to no coverage because it goes on too sheer and it is hard to apply. The Double Face Powder Foundation, is a pressed powder that contains talc and mineral oil; it can be used as an all-over sheer foundation or as a finishing powder, and the colors are so sheer it's really like wearing no makeup at all. Because of the mineral oil, I don't recommend Double

Face Powder for oily-skin types. Continuous Coverage Makeup ($12.50) is a very thick, heavy, opaque, oil-based foundation intended for those who want to cover scarring. It should not be used as an everyday makeup. The color selection is excellent and it is one of the better foundations of this type on the market for those who need this kind of coverage. It's not a look I recommend, however. ·

Foundation Colors to Try

Stay True Oil-Free ($14.50)
> Stay Beige: Great color.
> Stay Ivory: Great color.
> Stay Porcelain: May be too pink for some skin tones.
> Stay Sunny: Great color for tan skins.
> Stay Golden: Great color for dark skin tones and women of color.

Balanced Makeup Base ($11.50)
> Fair: Good color choice.
> Ivory: Great color.
> Warmer: Great color.
> Almond Beige: Good shade for women of color.

Extra Help ($18.50)
> Ivory Bisque: Good color choice.

Double Face Powder Foundation ($14.50)
> Matte Bisque: Great shade for fair skin tones.
> Matte Petal: Great shade for fair to medium skin tones.
> Matte Beige: Excellent color for fair to medium skin tones.
> Matte Honey: Great color for medium skin tones.
> Matte Tawny: Great color for tan skin tones.

Foundation Colors to Avoid

Balanced Makeup Base ($11.50)
> Honeyed Peach: This color is too orange for anyone's skin tone.
> Sun Glow: May be too orange for some skin tones.
> Honeyed Beige: Too orange, but may be worth a try.

Extra Help ($18.50)
> Fawn Beige: Too pink.
> Golden Almond: May turn orange.
> Amber Peach: Very orange for all skin tones.
> Beige Glow: Too orange for most skin tones.
> Copper Beige: May be too orange for most skin tones.

Double Face Powder Foundation ($14.50)
> Matte Ivory: Can be too peach for most skin types, but is so sheer that it may not matter.

Concealer: Clinique has an interesting assortment of concealers. Quick Corrector ($8.50) comes in a tube with a wand applicator; there are two shades, Light and Medium and both are excellent colors for light or medium skin tones. The texture is smooth without being greasy. Advanced Concealer ($10.50) comes in a squeeze tube and goes on like a liquid but dries to a powder. It comes in two shades, Light and Medium, and again both are excellent colors. This product is best for those with very smooth skin under the eye; any dry or rough skin will look worse when this type of concealer is placed over it. Clinique also has an Anti-Acne Control Formula Concealer ($10.50) that is very thick and heavy and comes in two shades, Light and Medium. The light is too pink and the Medium is too peach for most skin tones. The anti-acne part of the formula is colloidal sulfur and salicylic acid, ingredients that will not get rid of a blemish and can cause irritation.

Finishing Powder: Clinique has a loose powder ($14.50) that is talc-based and comes in a good selection of colors, and a transparent pressed powder ($11) that is also talc-based and comes in one shade that is supposed to be transparent; it didn't look that way when I applied it over my foundation.

Blush: Clinique has four types of blush: Soft Pressed Powder goes on very soft and slightly shiny (even the vivid colors go on sheer); Color Rub ($9.50) pours like a foundation out of a small bottle and spreads over the cheek or face like a very sheer liquid bronzer, but all the colors are shiny; Gel Rouge ($7.50), a liquid that comes in a tube and is to be rubbed over the cheek area to stain it with color — not a good idea for dry, oily or combination skin types, because it may tint open pores and flaky skin; and Creamy Blush, applied like a cream but dries to a powder, very sheer and all the colors are beautiful.

Blush Colors to Try
Powder Blush ($13.50)
> All of these color are beautiful: First Blush, Fig, Honey Blush, Plum Blush, Baby Rouge, Extra Clover, Extra Poppy, Pink Blush,

Rhubarb, Extra Violet, Extra Rose, New Clover, Lemon Geranium, Sun Duster and Powdered Light. Think Bronze and Chestnut Blush are both beautiful contour colors.

Creamy Blush ($9.50)
All of these colors are beautiful: Bronzed Rose, Warm Glow, Sunny Blush, Basic Blush, Honey Wine and Satin Mauve (which is very shiny, but may be good for evening wear).

Eyeshadow: Clinique makes three types of eyeshadow: Soft Pressed Eyeshadow goes on very soft and silky, but most of the shades are too shiny to recommend. Daily Eye Treat ($9.50) is a liquid in a tube. All the shades are very shiny, and the liquid dries in place, which makes blending tricky; Lid Sticks ($12.50) are fat pencils that come in mostly shiny colors. There are two soft, matte shades of peach and pink, Sunstone Flat and Blush Quartz.

Eyeshadow Colors to Try

Soft Pressed Eyeshadow ($10.50)
All of these are beautiful colors but slightly shiny: Pink Ginger, Blue Berry, Yellow Moon, Sun Ripe, Star Jade, Seashell Pink, Champagne, Ivory Bisque, Extra Violet, Charcoal, Brown Light, Brandied Plum, Gold Dust (very shiny, can be used for evening wear), Peach Silk and Blue Jade (as an accent color only).

Eyeshadow Colors to Avoid

Soft Pressed Eyeshadow ($10.50)
All of these colors are very shiny: Golden Lynx, Bronze Satin, Tea Leaf, Violet Rain, Sunset Mauve, Teal Haze, Earthling, Starstruck, Twilight Mauve, Starry Rose, Fawn Satin, Star Violet, Olive Bronze, and Silver Peony. Periwinkle Blue and Moon Turquoise are both too blue and too shiny.

Lipstick: Clinique has four types of lipstick that are all excellent choices. The color selection is wonderful and the textures are light but creamy. None of the selections provide matte or thick coverage — Different Lipstick ($9.50), Semi-Lipstick ($9.50), Super Lipstick (10.50) and Re-Moisturizing Lipstick ($9.50). I didn't notice large differences among the four types, although Semi-Lipstick was definitely greasier than the others; they are all worth a try.

Lip, Eye and Brow Pencils: Clinique's Lip Pencils ($9.50) have a soft, smooth texture and come in an excellent array of colors. There are two types of eye pencils: Regular Eye Pencils ($9.50) come in a good range of colors and go on soft, without a greasy feel; Quick Eyes ($13.50) has an eye pencil at one end of the stick and a powdered eyeshadow section with a sponge-tip applicator at the other. The eyeshadow is released into the sponge tip when you shake it. If the eyeshadow colors weren't so shiny, I would recommend this gimmicky product as a convenient tool for doing a fast eye design.

Mascara: Clinique's mascara ($11) is one of my favorites. It doesn't clump, smear or flake. The small brush is easy to control and builds color and length quickly and without a mess.

Cover Girl

When I approached the Cover Girl section of the drugstore, I was overwhelmed by the number of selections that loomed before me. This is was a huge array of products and colors. I gritted my teeth and began the process. The colors were bright and attractive, the packaging convenient and slick, and the variety of mascaras, blushes, eyeshadows, pressed powders and foundations impressive. When I unwrapped my cache at home, I encountered the problem with this line — overpowering fragrance. The odor was unmistakable; I think it's the same scent Cover Girl used when I was a teenager. If the odor doesn't bother you, Cover Girl has some wonderful blushes, pressed powders, lipsticks and a small selection of matte eyeshadows to consider. If not, this is line where the fragrance can get the better of you.

As is true with most cosmetics lines, the Cover Girl eyeshadow shades are more shiny than matte. There are various "types" of products in this line; for example there are six types of powder blushes in six assorted packages, but I found no discernible difference in how the colors go on or how they lasted, although most of the colors went on soft and sheer. The lipsticks are good, but in spite of the wide selection of mascaras I really only liked two of them. The line includes good large- and medium-size blush brushes that are worth considering if you don't have these essential applicators.

Cover Girl divides almost all of their colors into one of three color families; warm, cool and neutral. They provide a chart on the back of some of their products and most drugstores have a small computer-type device that helps you select your category. After you enter your hair color and skin color, it tells you what color family to select. This is a helpful, easy system to use, and their cool and warm categories are usually correct. However, they recommend that their neutral colors work with all skin tones and I would not agree with that.

Foundation: There are no testers available for Cover Girl foundations so I did not include them in this review. These foundations are highly fragranced and would be difficult to recommend even if there were testers. The Clarifying Makeup Foundation ($3.85), which is supposed to be used on acne-prone skin types contains salicylic acid, which is too drying and irritating and won't control acne.

Concealer: Cover Girl has several types of concealer. Their Clarifying Anti-Acne Concealer ($3.55) is basically a foundation in a tube that contains salicylic acid. Salicylic Acid won't get rid of acne and the colors of the foundation won't work on all skin tones. Moisturizing Concealer ($3.35) comes in four shades that are quite good and the consistency is creamy without being greasy. The All Day Perfecting Concealer ($3.55) is divided in half. One half is the concealer. The other (which looks like a lip gloss) is supposed to be a moisturizer. Sounds like a good idea, but it is an unnecessary step. Your moisturizer should take care of any dry skin under the eye and this "gloss" makes the undereye too greasy.

Finishing Powder: There are three types of pressed powder in the Cover Girl line that contain almost the same ingredients: Oil-Control Pressed Powder ($3.55) which contains talc, oat flour and mineral oil; Moisture Wear Pressed Powder ($3.50) which contains talc, mineral oil and oat flour; and Clean Makeup Pressed Powder ($3.25) which contains talc, kaolin, mineral oil and oat flour. They all come in a good selection of colors, but the way they are packaged makes it almost impossible to see the colors. They are also highly fragranced which makes them extremly difficult to recommend. The Oil-Control contains mineral oil which is not what you want to find in a product that should be oil-free.

Blush: Cover Girl has more blush types to choose from than any other line I reviewed. I didn't notice much of a difference between the ingredients in any of them or a difference in the way they went on. They are all talc-based with varying amounts of mineral oil and kaolin (clay). Some were too shiny — I don't recommend those and the fragrance was too sweet for my taste. But the colors were soft, went on well and lasted.

Blush Colors to Try

Cheekers ($2.25)

All of these colors are great: Rose Silk, Classic Pink, Snow Plum (slightly shiny) Pretty Peach, Crystal Plum, Soft Sable, Sunkissed Pink, Raspberries & Cream, Peaches & Cream, Watermelon Slice and Catalina Coral.

Soft Radiants ($3.75)

All of these colors are beautiful but go on very soft: Sweetheart Rose/Whispering Rose, Tawny Moon/New Moon, Wisteria/Wisteria Red, Wind Rose/Rose Mist, Sienna Sun/Sienna Sunbeam.

Classic Color Brush-On Blush ($3.55)

All of these colors are great: Natural Glow, Sun Warmed Coral, Fresh Peach and Plum Wine.

Replenishing Blush ($3.70)

All of these colors are great: Precious Plum, Pink Jasmine, Satin Rose, Sandalwood and Rose Petal.

Moisture Wear Blush ($4)

All of these colors are great: Empress Rose, Crystal Claret, Tender Peach, Plumberry, Cameo Pink and Morning Glow.

Blush Colors to Avoid

Cheekers ($2.25)

These colors are too shiny: Iced Ginger and Forever Heather.

Eyeshadow Colors to Try

Pro Colors ($2)

All of these colors are beautiful: Fawn, Dewy Pink (but can be too white for most skin tones), Marooned, Peach Nectar and Grey Suede (can be too blue).

Soft Radiants ($3.70)

All of these are beautiful matte colors: Soft Country Twilight, Soft Desert Blooms and Soft Forest Glade.

Eyeshadow Colors to Avoid

Pro Colors ($2)

All of these colors are extremely shiny: Mink, Tapestry Taupe, Rose Mist, Pink Chiffon, Whisper Blue (too blue), Buttercreme (too white), South Sea Blue, Magnolia, Snow Blossom (too white), Highland Heather (too blue), Moonlight, Autumn Haze, Ballet Pink, Khaki, Slate Blue (too blue), Silver Mist, Jade (too blue-green), Swiss Chocolate, Glazed Ginger, Milk & Honey and Champagne.

Soft Radiants ($3.70)

Soft Sky Lights: Too blue.
Soft Misty Morn: One shade is too blue.

Professional Color Match ($3.90/$5.40)

All of these colors are too shiny: Sante Fe Sunrise, Malibu Mist, Newport Twilight, Sonoma Sunset, Special Effects, Mountain Forest, Moody Mauves, Candlelight Dreams, Soft Focus, Ocean of Pearls (too blue) and Calypso Colors (difficult combination).

Luminese ($3.25)

All of these colors are too shiny: Shimmering Sands, Midnight Romance, Sparkling Wines, South Sea Breezes, Country Garden, Colorado Colors and Mediterranean Blue.

Lipstick: Cover Girl makes several types of lipstick. Their Continuous Color ($3.85) is a very creamy lipstick; Soft Radiants ($3.15), which is a somewhat glossy, sheer lipstick. Both are good and come in a small selection of excellent color choices. They also have a half powder, half gloss lip color combination called Lip Advance ($4.75) that causes much the same problems as all these products types do: They can tend to cake and lips become dried out after using these for an extended period of time.

Lip, Eye and Brow Pencils: Cover Girl has a full range of eyelining products that come in a small selection of colors: Prolining ($2.50) has a pencil on one end and a sponge-tip at the other but most of these colors have a slight shine; Eye Definer ($1.75) is a traditional pencil; Perfect Point Eye Pencil ($3.15) is an automatic pencil; Precision Liner ($4.45) is a felt-tip liquid liner; and Soft Liner ($3) is a traditional liquid liner. The liquid liners are always difficult for me to recommend and the pencils that aren't shiny or blue are fine, but it is hard to tell from the packaging exactly what color you are getting. You are fairly safe with colors like black and brown but that's about it. For those reasons I don't recommend most of the Cover Girl pencils.

Mascara: There are more types of Cover Girl mascaras than my eyelashes care to recall. None of these mascaras was particularly awful, but none of them was very good either. The variations were such that a couple of mascaras went on well but smudged; others went on poorly and didn't smudge; and then there were those that didn't go on well and also smudged. Not exciting and very disappointing.

Brushes: Cover Girl has two blush/powder brushes that are quite good. The large blush brush ($5.65) and the medium blush brush ($4.50) are both reliable and work well.

Elizabeth Arden

When I first started in the makeup business in the 1970s, Elizabeth Arden was the "old ladies line". The pink-and-white packaging was an age-old mainstay at the cosmetic counters, and indeed the line's clientele was almost exclusively women over 50. Now all that has changed and Elizabeth Arden competes well for the younger market.

The counter display is very attractive and easily accessible — always a strong point. The blush and lip colors are divided into four easy-to-understand categories: red tray, coral tray, pink tray and plum tray. There's enough color variety here to interest women of all skin tones. The eyeshadows are divided into two categories: cool and warm tones that are designed to coordinate with the blushes and lipsticks in the four color trays. Cool eyeshadows work with the pink or plum tray, and the warm eyeshadows work with the red and coral tray. Unfortunately, many of the eyeshadows are too shiny and should be avoided. The blush colors are attractive — none are shiny and almost all of them are worth a try.

Foundation: Elizabeth Arden has five types of foundation. Sponge-On Cream Makeup is extremely greasy and thick. The color choices are good, but for the most part, it is too heavy for me to recommend it to anyone. Simply Perfect Mousse Makeup is a unique foundation; it comes out like a foam and covers the face with a light, somewhat dry texture. The color selection is excellent, but it can take awhile to master the application technique. I tend to prefer traditional foundation consistencies and find this one a bit gimmicky. Flawless Finish Matte

Powder Makeup is a pressed powder, talc-based, that is recommended for use by itself as a foundation. It comes in a good range of colors, but I don't recommend powder as a foundation; it tends to look pasty and dull. But this can be used as a finishing powder. Arden's two liquid foundations are Flawless Finish Dewy Finish for normal to dry skin, and Flawless Finish Matte Finish for normal to oily skin, both of which have an excellent texture, but limited color choices.

Foundation Colors to Try

Flawless Finish Sponge-on Cream Makeup ($20)

Perfect Beige: Good color choice for light to medium skin tones.
Warm Beige: Good color choice for light to medium skin tones.
Toasty Beige: Great color for tan or medium skin tones.
Bronzed Beige: Great color for tan or deeper skin tones.

Simply Perfect Mousse Makeup ($17.50)

All of these colors are excellent (the shades are numbered from lightest to darkest): 4, 5, 6, 7, 8, 9, 10 and 11.

Flawless Finish Matte Powder Makeup ($20)

Honey Beige: Medium to dark skins tones only.
Luxury Beige: Medium to dark skins tones only.
Natural Tan: Medium to dark skins tones only.
French Bisque: Great color for lighter skin tones.

Flawless Finish Liquid Dewy Finish ($20)

All of these are excellent colors: French Bisque, Luxury Beige, Natural Tan and Warm Bronze.

Flawless Finish, Liquid Matte Finish ($20)

Perfect Ivory: Good color for fair skin tones, but may turn slightly pink on some skin tones.
Honey Beige: Good color, but can turn slightly peach on some skin tones.
French Bisque: Good color for medium skin tones.
Subtle Beige: Great color for tan skin tones.
Luxury Beige: Good color, but can turn slightly rose on some skin tones.
Natural Tan: Can be a good color, but may turn orange on some skin tones.
Warm Bronze: Can be a good color, but may turn orange on some skin tones.

Foundation Colors to Avoid

Flawless Finish Sponge-on Cream Makeup ($20)
 Porcelain Beige: Can turn slightly pink.
 Gentle Beige: Can turn slightly peach.
 Softly Beige: Can turn slightly peach.
 Toasty Rose: Can turn pink on most skin tones.
Simply Perfect Mousse Makeup ($17.50) ·
 All these colors can be too pink for most skin tones; 0,1,2 and 3.
Flawless Finish Matte Powder Makeup ($20)
 Perfect Ivory: Too pink for most skin tones.
 Cameo Creme: Too peach for most skin tones.
Flawless Finish Liquid Makeup, Dewy Finish ($20)
 Cameo Creme: Good color, but can turn peach.
 Honey Beige: Good color, but can turn peach.
 Subtle Beige: Too peach for most skin tones.
Flawless Finish Liquid Makeup, Matte Finish ($20)
 Cameo Creme: Too peach for most skin tones.

Concealer: Elizabeth Arden has two types of concealer. One in a traditional tube called Cream-On Concealer ($11) has a good consistency but is really too pink to use: A sheer Mousse Concealer comes in two shades that are also too pink. The Mousse Concealer is also difficult to use until you become accustomed to the squeeze top, and it does not provide the best texture for the job of concealing.

Finishing Powder: Elizabeth Arden's Flawless Finish Pressed Powder ($16) comes in three shades: Translucent Light, Translucent Medium and Translucent Dark. All contain talc and cornstarch and have light, sheer textures. There is also a a Bronzing Powder ($15) that comes in two shades: Golden Bronze is one of the nicest bronzing colors I've seen. It goes on soft, but there is always a problem with wearing a color that is intended to change and darken the color of your skin; and Pale Copper is too orange for anyone's skin tone.

Blush Colors to Try

Regular Blush ($16)
 All of these are great colors: Pink 3 (looks brighter then it goes
 on, good pink), Pink 2, Pink 1 (very soft plum), Plum 1, Plum 2,
 Plum 3, Neutral 1, Neutral 2, Neutral 3, Coral 1, Coral 2, Coral 3

and Cocoa 2 (great contour color). Also Fresh Corals and In The Pink (pretty, but both are too sheer for most skin tones).

Cream Powder Blush ($17.50)

All of these are great colors: Pink, Mauve, Coral, Mocha, and Cocoa which is a great contour color.

Eyeshadow Colors to Try

Singles, Duos, Trios and Quads ($12.50/$16/$20/$22.50)

Midnight Mauve/Moonlight Pink: Good color for darker skin tones.

Wild Violet/Lavender: Pretty combination.

Rhythm/Blue: Rhythm can look very, very pink.

Sophisticated Shadows: Lovely combination.

Misty Shadows: Very subtle combination of grays.

Moonscape Shadows: For evening wear only.

Gold Lit Shadows: For evening wear only.

Horizons: Probably for dramatic looks only.

Fresco Shadows: Very soft and pretty combination for fair skin tones.

Vintage Shadows: Definitely worth a try.

Almond/Slate: Great combination.

The Classics: Beautiful combination.

Sea Glass: Fairly bright and sheer.

Eyeshadow Colors to Avoid

Singles, Duos, Trios and Quads ($12.50/$16/$20/$22.50)

Wild Grape/Citrus: Difficult combination and shiny.

Haze/Blue diamond: Too blue for anyone.

Art Deco Shadows: Difficult combination to use.

Daybreak Shadows: Difficult combination to use.

Jade/Pink Lotus: Awkward combination.

Teakwood/Silver: Too shiny.

Aegean Blue/Caribbean Blue: Too blue and too green.

Bittersweet/Heather/Heather Mist: Too shiny.

Sunlight/Pink Champagne: Very yellow and pink and too shiny.

Fresh Lilac Shadows: Too shiny.

Highland Shadows: The colors are too contrasting and bright.

Tradewinds: Difficult combination of colors and very blue.

Sandswept: Too sheer; it would take a lot of product to show.

Lipstick: Both types of lipstick are easily accessible for testing and are divided into extremely helpful color groupings of plum, pink, coral and red. Luxury Lipsticks ($12) go on somewhat sheer and moist and they provide light coverage. Moisture Lipsticks ($12) feel very greasy and more like a gloss than a lipstick. Elizabeth Arden makes a product called Lip Fix ($12) that is supposed to prevent lipstick from feathering into the lines around the mouth. It works well for most but not all lipsticks, and I don't care for the squeeze-tube applicator. Lip Fix goes on like a moisturizer and must dry before you put on your lipstick. For touch ups during the day, it isn't the best. I prefer anti-feathering products that come in lipstick form.

Eye, Brow and Lip Pencils: Elizabeth Arden has a beautiful array of both eye and lip pencil colors called Slender Liners ($9). Some of the colors are wonderful. If you do consider these pencils, be sure to avoid Peacock and Emerald, both of which are too green for most eyes. There is also a liquid felt-tip eyeliner called Luxury Eyeliner Pen ($15). It goes on smoothly and evenly but doesn't blend and tends to look too much like a line. Nevertheless, the product's good for a dramatic eye design or for those who can't use pencils without having them smudge. The Brow Powders ($11) are applied with brushes and come in workable shades. Soft Blonde and Sable are great colors, though an ash/brown shade would be helpful. I prefer applying eyebrow color with eyeshadow powders or powders designed specifically for the eyebrow because it looks so much softer and more natural than pencil color. Be careful not to make it look like a line by putting it on too heavily. It is best to use a soft brush — not the hard one that Elizabeth Arden packages with the Brow Powder. All the pencils in this line have a good texture, but nothing unique, like almost all the other pencils on the market.

Mascara: For the most part, I like Elizabeth Arden's mascaras. They go on well, don't clump and don't smear. The only problem product is their Two Brush Mascara ($12), which has two shapes of brushes at each end of the mascara tube. The idea sounds good — one shape does the job of putting the mascara on, the other is supposed to lengthen and separate — but I didn't notice a real difference between the two sides. I did notice, however, that this mascara dried up faster than others. Two brushes pumping air into the same tube would make any mascara become dry faster than usual.

Estee Lauder

Estee Lauder is the grande dame of makeup lines. Ask any of the women who work the counters for this well respected, veteran cosmetics company and they will tell you the products sell themselves. The sales at Lauder counters exceed those at just about all of the other cosmetics lines. Because Estee Lauder is so successful, they command a large amount of counter space at most department stores. What does Estee Lauder do so well? Perhaps advertising is the key here. For years they marketed their products as elegant but fresh — for the classic girl or woman next door. Then, as the fashion changed, they changed their marketing direction and placed the emphasis on sophistication and glamour. I guess the fresh look is nice but not very distinct. They also have a very well trained, loyal sales force. Do the products live up to the new image (or the old image, for that matter)? Some of the products are ok, but I can't say that they are outstanding, and some of the products in this line are difficult to use.

A select number of stores have private makeup areas and skin analyzing machines that are really quite impressive. The counter displays are not accessible without the help of a salesperson. For the most part, the eyeshadows are either too shiny or too intense for day-time wear, although the intense shades are great for women of color. The foundations are excellent. I particularly like the Demi-Matte and the Fresh Air, but you need to be careful about color choice; there are many pink and orange foundations in this collection. Most of the blushes are lovely, but mostly for women with darker skin tones, although they do have a small selection of softer colors that are good for lighter skin tones.

Foundation: Estee Lauder has six types of foundation, all of which are quite good: Demi-Matte is a superior oil-free foundation; Fresh Air (for normal to oily skin) has a lovely finish but exceptionally poor color choices; Country Mist is recommended for normal to dry skin and provides an excellent medium-coverage foundation for dry skin, though I don't recommend it for normal-skin types; Polished Performance (for dry skin) gives a sheer, more natural coverage and is an excellent liquid foundation for normal and dry skin types, although the colors all have a rose tint that is a problem a for most skin tones; Sportswear Tint is almost like wearing no makeup, but it does contain a Sun Protecting Factor of 12 (15 would be better); and ReNutriv (for very dry skin) provides fairly heavy coverage which is probably too heavy for any skin type. All of the Lauder foundations are divided into golden, neutral and pink shades, and are then rated 1 to 4 for light to fair skin tones. The rating system is helpful, but always avoid foundations with pink tones.

Foundation Colors to Try

Fresh Air Makeup ($17.50)

Palm Beige: Worth a try for darker or tan skin tones.

Linen Beige: Good color for fair skin tones.

Cloud Beige: Good color for fair skin tones.

Nutmeg Brown: Great shade for women of color.

Honey Pecan: For women of color only, but may turn orange.

Demi-Matte ($19.50)

Fresh Beige: Good medium shade, but may turn slightly rose on some skin tones.

Champagne Beige: Great color.

Wheat Beige: Great medium color tone, but may be too yellow for some skin tones.

Rose Beige: Good medium color tone, but may turn slightly rose on some skin tones.

Natural Ivory: Great color for fair skin tones.

Golden Beige: Good medium color, but may be too yellow for some skin tones.

Ivory Beige: Good color for fair to medium skin tones.

Sun Bronze: Excellent color for darker skin tones.

Polished Performance ($25)

All of these colors are acceptable, but they all tend to turn rose: Perfect Beige, Outdoor Beige, Cool Beige, Wild Honey, Alabaster Beige, Vanilla Mist, Blushing Beige, Summer Beige, Tender Rose Beige, and Sunlit Beige. Butternut Bronze and Tawny Almond are both great golden colors for darker skin tones.

Country Mist Liquid ($17.50)

Suntan Beige: Beautiful tan color.

Golden Beige: Beautiful color for medium skin tones.

Clear Beige: Beautiful color for medium skin tones.

Warm Beige: Great color for medium skin tones.

Misty Tan: Good color, but may turn slightly rose on some skin tones.

Tender Beige: Good color for fair skin tones.

Beige Light: Great color for fair to medium skin tones.

Vanilla Beige: Great color for fair to medium skin tones.

Sportswear Tint ($25)

All of these are excellent colors: Light Tint, Bronze Tint and Golden Tint.

Foundation Colors to Avoid

Fresh Air Makeup ($17.50)

Ivory Mist: May be too pink for most skin tones.

Meadow Beige: May be too ashy or green.

Beige Glow: May be too pink.

Newport Beige: May be too pink.

Sunrise Beige: Too orange.

Warm Beige: Too orange.

Demi-Matte Liquid ($19.50)

Rose Ivory: Too pink for most skin tones.

Country Mist Liquid ($17.50)

Morning Beige: Too peach for most skin tones.

Country Beige: Too rose for most skin tones.

Concealer: Estee Lauder's concealer ($12.50) comes in three shades: Light, Medium and Barely Mauve. The light is fairly pink, the medium is good and the barely mauve is a white-lavender shade. The consistency is on the dry side. I wouldn't give this concealer high marks, but it isn't awful either.

Finishing Powder: Estee Lauder has two types of powder: Demi-Matte for oily skin is talc-based; and Lucidity Translucent Loose Powder. ($25) for all skin types. Lucidity is a new product that is promoted to change the way light focuses on your face. It felt good, but I saw no real difference on my skin from other powders I've used. Demi-Matte has a great texture, but most of the color choices go on too chalky. The Moisture Balanced Face Powder has been discontinued.

Finishing Powder Colors to Try

Demi-Matte Face Powder ($18.50)

Medium: Not really a medium shade, but it is good for fair skin tones.

Dark: Will go on chalky for dark or tan skin tones.

Finishing Powder Colors to Avoid
Demi-Matte Face Powder ($18.50)
Light: Will go on too white and pink for almost all skin tones.
Pink Tint: Will go on too white and pink for almost all skin tones.
Sunlight: Too white.

Concealer: Estee Lauder used to have two different concealers, but they discontinued the Cream Concealer just before this book went to press. It was too greasy for all but extremely dry skin, and even then it was likely to set into the lines around the eye, which is probably why it was suspended. The Automatic Cream Concealer ($12.50) comes in a tube and has a slightly dry consistency which makes it somewhat difficult to recommend for dry skin. The color choices are problematic: Light may be too pink for most skin tones; Medium is good only for darker skin tones; and Barely Mauve blends to a whitish pink that may be too pink for most skin tones.

Blush: Estee Lauder has two kinds of blusher: Signature Powder has a nice array of colors but several are somewhat shiny, although not excessively so; Soft Color Creme Blush goes on like a cream and dries on the skin like a powder. It has a beautiful consistency and is great for normal to oily skin.

Blush Colors to Try
Signature Powder Blush ($20)
Crystal Rose: Very pink, but goes on softly.
Rose Fawn: Good color.
Blushing: A good, soft coral tone.
Nut Brown Apple: Good contour color.
Cranberry Mist: Soft pretty plum tone.
Avant Red: For dark or tan skin only.
Brandied Rose: For dark or tan skin only.
Fire: Too orange for most skin tones, good for dark skin tones.
Claret: For dark skin tones only.
Just Blush: Beautiful, soft blush color and no shine.
Pink Blush: Beautiful, soft blush color and no shine.
Ginger Blush: Beautiful, soft blush color and no shine.
Peach Blush: Beautiful, soft blush color and no shine.

Soft Color Creme Blush ($20)
All of these are beautiful colors: Red Silk, Rose Velvet, Sienna Suede, Pink Cashmere and Peach Chiffon (although it may be too orange for most skin tones).

Eyeshadow Colors to Try
Singles, Duos and Trios ($15/$20/$25)
Soft Peach: Good peach color, but slightly shiny.
Plumberry: Great brown color, but slightly shiny.
Mercury: Beautiful gray and no shine.
Blue Enamel/Grey Smoke/Crystal: Good colors, but can be a tricky combination to use.
Slate/Azalea/Sunflower: Good colors, but may be a tricky combination to use.
Coffee/Peach Cream/Ivory Cream: Great combination of colors, though too shiny for daytime wear.
Coal/Chamois/Brownstone: Great neutral color combination, though slightly shiny.
Pink Mist/Warm Walnut: Combination of colors may be difficult to use but the individual colors are good for dark skin tones.
Alabaster/Mushroom: Good colors though Alabaster may be too white for most skin tones.
Antique Gold/Plum Perfect: Shiny colors but may be good for evening wear.
Pistachio/Pink Blaze: Difficult color combination but may be good for evening wear.

Eyeshadow Colors to Avoid
Singles, Duos and Trios ($15/$20/$25)
All these colors are too shiny: Anthracite, Sea Pearl Beige, Sterling, Highlight Pink, Camellia/Sunbeam/Pink Shine, Plum Wine/Grape/Pale Peach, Cobalt/Limelight/Cerulean (shiny and a difficult combination of colors to use), Amethyst Sea/Misty Lilac/Blue Moon, Nectarine/Forest, Lilac Sky/Twilight, Misty Aqua/Twilight Teal (only slightly shiny, but definitely too blue) and Blue Haze/Smoke.

Lipstick: Estee Lauder has four types of lipstick: Perfect Lipstick ($15), All Day Lipstick ($12), Feather Proof ($12) and Polish Performance ($12). The Perfect Lipstick and All Day Lipstick are by far the best and definitely worth a try. The Feather Proof and Polish Performance lipsticks will probably be discontinued shortly. Neither has a great consistency, and the Feather Proof is not feather-proof. Many of the salespeople I talked to don't recommend them and I agree.

Eye, Brow and Lip Pencils: Estee Lauder's Signature Liners ($22.50) for the lips, brows and eyes are automatic pencils that come in an elegant container. They are among the most expensive pencils on the market, and except for the container, they are not unusual or special. Unlike other automatic pencils, they roll up as well as down, so you don't have to worry about sharpening or wasting. Some of the eye pencils are too shiny and fairly greasy.

Mascara: Estee Lauder's More Than Mascara ($15) goes on easily while building nice thick lashes without clumping. Unfortunately, when I washed my face the mascaras burned my eyes. How disappointing when the mascara went on so beautifully.

Specialty Products: Estee Lauder's Brow Gel ($12.50) comes in clear and a handful of other shades that can make the brow look thick and keep it in place. This is a definite consideration for those who want a thicker, but soft-looking brow, without the definition of a pencil.

Fashion Fair

For women of color and African-American women, Fashion Fair is a wonderful, complete line of products with a superior assortment of colors. There are many other options available for women of color, but for the widest selection possible, particularly in lipsticks, foundations, blushes and concealing creams, this line, though not perfect, is nevertheless outstanding. One major downfall needs to be mentioned: almost all of Fashion Fair eyeshadows are intensely shiny. I don't recommend shiny eyeshadow for women of color any more than I do for women with lighter skin tones. Shiny eyeshadows make eyelids look wrinkly, and they are always inappropriate in daytime. However, Fashion Fair has a line of fragrance-free products that are worth looking at. There are two types of oil-free foundations, blushes, concealer creams and lipsticks. There is also a selection of products that contain fragrance, and these, too, are good quality. The display units are all easily accessible and the saleswomen I met seemed generally well trained and helpful.

Foundation: Fashion Fair has five types of foundation: Oil-Free Souffle is fragrance-free, applies with a wet sponge, and goes on like a pancake foundation. It can be tricky to use, but the color selection and coverage are excellent (although it may look somewhat pasty on normal-to-dry skin). Oil-Free Liquid is an excellent foundation with great color selection for normal-to-oily skin. Liquid Sheer Foundation works best on dry skin, and there is a superior array of colors. Perfect Finish Creme Makeup is a compact foundation that is fairly greasy, which may cause the foundation color to turn orange. Foundations for women of color, and women with darker skin tones in particular, contain more pigment, and the oil intensifies the pigment.

Foundation Colors to Try

Oil-Free Souffle ($20)
> All these colors are superior: Beige Glo, Amber Glo, Honey Glo, Tawny Glo, Copper Glo, Tender Glo, Brown Blaze Glo, Bronze Glo, Pure Brown Glo, Ebony Glo and Pure Pearl Glo, which may turn slightly pink on some skin tones.

Oil-Free Liquid ($16.50)
> All these colors are superior: Beige, Honey Amber, Tender Brown, Copper Blaze, Bare Bronze, Ebony Brown.

Perfect Finish Creme Makeup ($16.50)
> Beige Glo: Great color choice.
> Tender Glo: Great color, but can be slightly ashy on some skin tones.
> Brown Blaze Glo: Good color, but may turn orange on some skin tones.
> Bronze Glo: Good color, but may turn orange on some skin tones.
> Ebony Glo: Great color for ebony skin tones.

Liquid Sheer Foundation ($11.50)
> All these colors are beautiful: Alabaster, Beige, Toffee Tone, Honey Amber, Tender Brown, Copper Blaze, Bare Bronze, Ebony Brown.

Foundation Colors to Avoid

Oil-Free Liquid ($16.50)
> Toffee Tone: Can be too yellow for most skin tones.
> Tawny: Can be too yellow for most skin tones.
> Copper Tan: Can be too orange for most skin tones.

Perfect Finish Creme Makeup ($16.50)
Pure Pearl Glo: Can be too pink for most skin tones.
Amber Glo: Can be too yellow for most skin tones.
Honey Glo: Can be too yellow for most skin tones.
Tawny Glo: Can be too orange for most skin tones.
Copper Glo: Can be too orange for most skin tones.
Liquid Sheer Foundation ($11.50)
Tawny: Can be too yellow on most skin tones.
Copper Tan: Can turn orange on some skin tones.

Concealer: Fashion Fair has three types of concealer. Cover Tone Concealing Creme ($12) is for use under the eyes or over blemishes and scars. It has a very dry consistency and provides fairly heavy coverage. It is supposed to be used with a Setting Powder ($12). The saleswoman told me the powder was waterproof, but all it contains is talc with some preservative. I don't recommend the Concealing Creme or the Setting Powder. The other two concealers are excellent. Fragrance-Free Coverstick has a drier consistency for oily skin; the other Coverstick has fragrance and a creamier formula. All the shades are fabulous and definitely worth a try.

Concealer Colors to Try
Fragrance-Free Coverstick ($9)
All of these colors are excellent: Very Light, Light, Medium, and Dark.
Fragrance Coverstick ($9)
All of these colors are excellent: Very Light, Light, Medium, and Dark.

Finishing Powder: Fashion Fair has a loose powder ($14.50) and a pressed powder ($11); both contain talc and mineral oil. They have good texture and an excellent range of colors.

Blush: Fashion Fair has a wonderful variety of blush colors both fragranced and fragrance-free. They go on smooth and include vivid and subtle shades. This is an excellent assortment to consider, although some of the colors have too much shine to be really suitable for daytime.

Blush Colors to Try

Fragrance-Free ($12)

Rich Ruby: Great color choice.

Terra Rose: Too shiny, but may be good for evening wear.

Russian Sable: This is a very shiny brown blush, but may be good for an evening wear contour shade.

Metallic Mauve: Beautiful color.

Honey Topaz: Great color.

Brandy Mist: Good mauve-brown shade.

Fragranced ($12)

All of these colors are beautiful, but fairly shiny: Paradise Pink, Plum Pearl, Fiesta Pink, Rasberry Ice, Crystal Rose, Moonlit Mauve, Chocolate Chip, Quiet Coral, Pearly Paprika, Plum Rose (only slightly), Royal Red, Plum Rich, Wild Plum, Ginger Berry, Crimson, Bronze (an excellent contour color) and Golden Lights a beautiful bronze highlighter for evening.

Eyeshadow: As I've said, all of the Fashion Fair eyeshadows are extremely shiny. They are not the best option for women of color. The two shades of brown that aren't shiny each come packaged in a set of four colors, and the other three are shiny. I do not recommend any of the Fashion Fair eyeshadows except possibly for evening wear.

Eyeshadow Colors to Avoid

Singles, Duos, Trios, Quads and Quints ($12.50 to $14.50)

All of these colors are extremely shiny: Winter Berry/Golden, Chestnut, Classy Copper/Golden Nectar, Wild Orchid/Caribbean Blue, Frost Rose/Satin Brown, Silver Light, Midnight Blue, Golden Glow, Lavender Beauty, Misty Brick, Black Pearl, Smoky Emerald, Rich Plum, Shades of Mardi Gras I, Shades of Mardi Gras II, Shades of Mardi Gras III, Shades of Fantasy I, Shades of Fantasy II, Shades of Fantasy III. Shades of Beauty I and Shades of Beauty II both have shiny shadows except for one in each.

Lipstick: Since the range of shades appropriate for women of color is so extensive, it would be nice if Fashion Fair's lipsticks ($19.50) were more creamy and less greasy.

Lancome

Lancome is one of the more popular cosmetics lines. The prices are steep, but relatively reasonable given Lancome's place at the high end of the cosmetics range. The product line is impressively varied and many of the items were well liked by most of the women who responded to my survey. This French line is very low-key and maintains a more casual air than the other French lines sold at the department stores. The Lancome saleswomen seemed to be cooperative and helpful without being haughty or condescending. This line seems to attract women interested in a conservative makeup look, even though some of its colors are too shiny and vivid to facilitate that kind of image — so be careful. I like the Lancome display units very much. They are accessible and easy to use, particularly if you want to experiment on your own. I do wish, however, that Lancome would follow the trend of the other makeup lines and divide their blushes, eyeshadows, lipsticks and lipliners into color groups.

I was disappointed to find that many of Lancome's eyeshadow colors are extremely bright and shiny. There are at least five types of eyelining products, but some of the eye pencil colors are also too intense and shiny. They would encourage women to make a mistake I see frequently — overlined eyes. Lancome's waterproof pencils are fat and difficult to sharpen and I don't recommend them. There also are two types of liquid liners that I don't recommend unless you are looking for an obvious "lined" look.

Lancome's lipstick colors are wonderful, though the company's promise of long-lasting lipstick (it claims five hours with its new one) just didn't pan out. The blush colors, particularly the new cream powder blush called Blush Majeur, are for the most part soft and quite pretty. Lancome has some of the best color choices available in foundations; almost all of them are great shades without any pink or orange tones. Prepackaged testers are available from time to time, which makes trying on makeup much easier than using a cotton swab and cotton balls. If Lancome ever gets an assortment of matte eyeshadows, reduces the intense color of some of their eye pencils and updates their tester units, this would be one of the most reliable cosmetics lines.

Foundation: Lancome has quite an array of foundations to choose from: Maquivelour (for normal to dry skin) has a soft light texture with even coverage. Maquicontrole is the ultimate oil-free foundation; it goes on dry and can stay that way for awhile, which is great for extremely oily skin, but it can also be very thick and heavy and difficult to blend. Creme Compact Makeup has a creamy feel but goes on like a powder. It has a wonderful texture and glides over the face beautifully, but like most of the new foundations, it is best for combination or normal skin. Dual Finish ($24) has ingredients more like a compact powder than a foundation. It comes in an excellent assortment of colors and can be used wet, although I think it tends be too powdery when used by itself. It makes a great finishing powder.

Foundation Colors to Try

Maquicontrole ($26)
> Champagne Beige: Great color for fair skin.
> Pale Beige: Great color for fair skin.
> Buffed Bisque: Great color for light skin.
> Shell Beige: Great color for light to medium skin.
> Honey Beige: Great shade for women of color.

Maquivelour ($27)
> All of these are great colors: Truly Beige, Beige Bisque, Softly Tan, Sun Bisque and Desert Beige.

Creme Compact Makeup ($26)
> Creme d'Ivoire: Great for fair skin tones.
> Rose Pale Beige: Can go on slightly pink.
> Peche Buff: Can be too green on some skin tones.
> Tres Beige: Great tan color.
> Beige Soliel: Great tan color.

Foundation Colors to Avoid

Maquicontrole ($26)
> Soft Cameo: Too pink.
> Blushed Beige: Too pink.
> Caramel: Can look ashen on African-American skin tones.

Maquivelour ($27)
> Porcelaine: Too pink.
> Beige Sand: Too pink.
> Peach Cream: Too pink.
> Beige Cream: Too ashy for most skin tones.
> Rose Buff: Too orange.
> Warm Beige: May be too ashy for most skin tones.
> Beige Honey: May be too orange for most skin tones.

Creme Compact Makeup ($26)
   Beige Amande: Can go on too orange for most skin types.
   Rose Clair: Can be too rose for most skin types.

Concealer: Lancome makes a waterproof eyeshadow base simply called Shadow Base ($12.50). It is quite waterproof, which means it must be removed with an oil-based cleanser, but because of its color and consistency, it nicely tones down the intense shine of Lancome's iridescent eyeshadows and eyeshadow pencils. However, I never recommend doing two things when you can do one, so it's best to forget the shadow base and instead use foundation on your lid and wear eyeshadows that are matte, not shiny. Besides, I found no difference in how long my eyeshadow lasted when I wore Shadow Base instead of foundation. For covering dark circles under the eye, Anti-Cernes ($12.50) comes in three shades — Light, Medium and Dark. It is a waterproof coverup that goes on creamy but dries to a somewhat powdery, matte finish. I'm not fond of this concealer. I have noticed, and several of the Lancome salespeople have too, that the cream fills in the lines around the eye, the colors are bit too pink or peach for most skin tones, and the tube applicator is hard to control, particularly when the product is almost gone and you have to squeeze a little harder so you can use it all.

Finishing Powder: Lancome has three shades of pressed powders ($22). They go on smoothly without a chalky finish and the colors Translucent and Matte Beige are excellent; Matte Peche is too peach for most skin tones. Lancome also has a loose powder called Poudre Majeur ($24) which is a very good powder made without talc; it contains clay and zinc instead. All the colors are quite good — Ivoire, Sand, Bisque, Rose, Honey, Bronze and Buff. It also claims to have "micro-bubbles." Whatever that means, it's still only a powder.

Blush: Blush Majeur is a cream blush with a beautiful consistency. It's worth trying if you want a soft blush look, but only if you can handle the blending. Maquiriche is a traditional blush; the texture is smooth and velvety and the colors go on soft.

Blush Colors to Try
Blush Majeur ($19)
   All of these colors are beautiful: Petunia, Rose, Berry, Sienna, Hibiscus, Red, Tulip, Sepia and Mocha (a great contour color).

Maquiriche ($18.50)
All of these are good colors: Corail Douce, Matte Rouge, Gilded Bronze, Cedar Rose, Camille, Pink Soleil (may be too bright for fair skin tones), Aplum (probably too shiny for most skin tones), Raspberry (good color for dark skin tones) and Rose Ivoire.

Eyeshadow: This is the weakest link in an otherwise good product line. I do not recommend most of the eyeshadows because the colors are either too shiny or in a difficult combination to use.

Eyeshadow Colors to Try
Singles, Duets and Quartettes ($16/$20/$24)
Country Heather: Could look reddish on pale skin tones.
Muscat: Good eyeliner color or shading for the back corner of the eye.
Lezard: Good eyeliner color or shading for the back corner of the eye, though slightly shiny.
Ambre: Great color for blondes and redheads, but slightly shiny.
Flume de Terre: Good medium shades.
Harmonique Sepia: Great color combination, but slightly shiny.
Couleurs Boheme: Great color combination, but slightly shiny.
Symphonie d'Automne: Great color combination, but very shiny, for evening wear only.
Coutoure de Lancome: *Wonderful* color combination and not shiny.

Eyeshadow Colors to Avoid
Singles, Duets and Quartettes ($16/$20/$24)
All of these colors are too shiny: Cafe au Lait, Nosegay, Silversmoke/Fawn, French Cream (can be too white), Cari, Les Charades, Lavandou/Violette (Lavandou is very shiny), Peche/Raisin, Tiara/Operetta, Bronze Mica/Golden Sun, Peach Cire/Goldspun Smoke, Tiara, Alfresco, Nuit Dore, Rose Dore, White Gold, Golden Leaf, Les Imaginaire, Etoile de Nuit, Fanfare Lancome, Fete Frolique, Printemps, Parasol Exotique, Couleurs Savage (great combination for evening wear only), Potpourri (great combination of colors, evening wear only), Soiree Noel (difficult combination of colors), Pink Ivory/Organdy (difficult combination of colors to use) and Nuance Mystere (only one of the shades).

Lipstick: Lancome's lipsticks are mostly very good and the colors are lovely. The Maquiglace Le Stylo ($14) is more like a gloss than a lipstick and won't last very long. They used to have a lip-coloring pen called Pinceau Rouge that was extremely difficult to use and has been discontinued; so much for that gimmick. They have also discontinued Maquiglace and Rouge a Levres. The lipsticks that remain are Hydra-Riche ($14) and a new one, Rouge Superb ($15). Both are worth checking out, though none of the claims about long-lasting color or reduced feathering were confirmed.

Lipliner: Lancome has an automatic lip pencil called Le Crayon ($12) that never needs sharpening. It's convenient to use, though a bit expensive for what you get, since there is no real difference between this and a regular pencil you have to sharpen.

Eye Pencil: Le Crayon Khol ($11) is the name for Lancome's eyelining pencils. They are good (though not exceptional) and come in a nice range of colors, but they are no better then others I've found on the market for less money. The claim that they don't smudge once they're on is not entirely accurate; smudging is caused by several factors, not just the pencil itself. They also make a waterproof pencil called Le Crayon ($12.50). There are over 15 colors to choose from, but most are shiny, though some of the darker shades like brown and black are not, and they are fairly waterproof. I find this product difficult to recommend for several reasons: first it is hard to get off without using a wipeoff makeup remover, and I would never suggest doing that; it is hard to sharpen; and the darker colors are more waterproof than the lighter colors and none of them is 100 percent waterproof, which means they come off unevenly while you are in the water. There are also two types of liquid liners, Maquiglace Liquid Liner ($13) and an Eyelining Felt Pen ($18.50). Both make very definite lines that do not blend. This can be good for some eye designs, but I don't often recommend such an obvious look. If you like it, the felt pen is definitely an interesting way to put on eyeliner.

Brow Pencil: I do not recommend Brow Pencil ($13.50) for eyebrows because penciled brows look artificial and out of date — way out of date. But if you are used to wearing pencil on your brows and can't imagine doing it any other way, this is a good pencil to consider. It has a brush at one end so that you can feather the color as you apply it, to keep the brow from looking like a harsh line. Of course you can get the same effect by using almost any eyebrow pencil and brushing the brow with an old toothbrush or brow brush — just as effective and cheaper. The Taupe color, however, is too shiny for anyone to try, and Brunette can be too red for many skin tones.

Mascara: Lancome makes reliable mascaras ($13.50) that usually don't smudge and are very popular. There are six different types. I found that the Immencils and Keracils tended to clump, but they did make the lashes very thick, almost too thick. The others were just fine and are worth a try.

Brushes: Lancome is one of the few lines at the department stores that sell a somewhat reasonably priced set of brushes ($32). These aren't exceptional and there are cheaper ones elsewhere, but they are reliable and the bests way to apply makeup.

L'Oreal

It is fitting that L'Oreal follows Lancome in my alphabetical listing, because both are owned by the same parent company in France. This is a good drugstore line and I feel confident about recommending many of their products, although the selections are somewhat limited. Since some drugstore lines have an overwhelming array of products, it isn't necessarily a negative that L'Oreal's collection is smaller than most. As is true of most eyeshadows in most lines, their colors are too shiny to recommend. Their foundations have a smooth texture, but do not have the best color selections (several are too pink or orange). But there are a few excellent shades of Mattique Oil-Free Foundation that are worth checking out. L'Oreal's other products, however, are outstanding. You won't be disappointed with their blushes, lipsticks, powders or mascaras. The blush colors, both the regular blush and the cream powder blush, have a beautiful texture and are some of the best around. There are three types of lipsticks in this line and the colors, wearability, textures and consistency are all fabulous. I would rate L'Oreal's mascaras as some of the best on the market for the money.

Foundation: L'Oreal is one of the few drugstore lines to make foundation tester units available. What a plus! An inexpensive foundation is no bargain if you buy the wrong color.

Foundation Colors to Try

Mattique ($7.50, oil-free)

> Beige Blush: Good color for medium skin tones, but can turn peach.
>
> Nude Beige: Excellent color for fair to medium skin tones.
>
> Buff Beige: Excellent color for fair skin tones.
>
> Sand Beige: Excellent color for fair to medium skin tones.
>
> Honey Beige: Good color for medium to dark skin tones, but may turn orange.
>
> Rich Beige: Excellent tan color.

Visuelle ($7.50, normal to dry skin)

> Bare Beige: Good color for fair skin tones.
>
> Deep Beige: Could be a good tan color, but may turn rose on some skin tones.

Foundation Colors to Avoid

Mattique ($7.50, oil-free)

> Soft Ivory: Too pink for most skin tones.
>
> Golden Beige: Too orange for most skin tones.

Visuelle ($7.50, normal to dry skin)

> Ivory: Too pink for most skin tones.
>
> Palest Beige: Too peach for most skin tones.
>
> Sand Beige: Too pink for all skin tones.
>
> Pink Beige: Too orange for all skin tones.
>
> Bisque: Too orange.
>
> Honey: Too orange.

Finishing Powder: L'Oreal has four shades of pressed powders ($7.50). They have a sheer finish but contain wheatstarch, which can cause allergic reactions in some people. The colors are quite attractive. Transparence Light may be too white for most tones; Transparence Light-Medium, Medium and Transparence Deep are all wonderful colors.

Blush: L'Oreal makes two kinds of blush, one a regular blush with a gorgeous texture called Visuelle, and another called Micro Blush. Micro Blush goes on like a cream and dries to a powder, gives very soft coverage and has great staying powder. The only negative is that like most of the cream-to-powder blushes it can be tricky to use.

Blush Colors to Try

Visuelle Powder Blush ($7.25)

All these are gorgeous colors: Plume, Tulipe, Fraiche, Capucine, Rose, Peony Pink, Rouge Russet and Cameo (excellent contour color).

Micro Blush ($7.25)

All these are gorgeous colors: Champagne Rose, Tres Pink, Mauvesse, Creme Bordeaux, Pink Delight, Camellia, Terre Rose and Brunelle (beautiful contour color).

Eyeshadow Colors to Avoid

Trios and Quads ($4.25)

All of these colors are beautiful, but too shiny to recommend: Bleu, Plume, Earth, Gris, Rose, Gold Rust, Purple Pink, Desert Stone, Terre Peach, Rose Plum, Fantome (difficult combination), Taupe Peche, Teal, Cafe and Violette.

Lipstick: L'Oreal makes three types of lipstick: Colour Supreme ($5.75), Creme Riche ($5.25) and L'Artiste Creme ($5.50). All are quite creamy, have a wonderful texture and last slightly longer than average. They rival any lipstick you will find at department store cosmetics counters. I didn't find any significant differences among the three types of lipstick; they all went on, looked and felt pretty much the same, which is great if you're looking for a good creamy, fairly matte lipstick.

Eye Pencil: L'Oreal has a good selection of pencils called Le Grand Kohl ($4.50). Most of these colors are fairly muted, go on smooth without being greasy, and blend easily without streaking.

Mascara: I found both of L'Oreal's mascaras to be excellent, but I particularly liked the Formula Riche ($4.95) and would consider buying it again and again. It did not smear, it separated the lashes nicely without making them look spiked or clumped and the wand was easy to use. I also very much liked the Lash Out Mascara ($4.95), but I prefer a shorter wand; other than that it is an excellent product. Formula Riche contains more mascara than Lash Out, so it is by far the better buy.

Mary Kay

Of all the lines I shopped, I knew the least about Mary Kay's products and, to be honest, I expected the worst. I had read my share about the beauty dynasty that Mary Kay Ash and her son had built. Although I was skeptical about their home makeup demonstrations, I used the Yellow Pages to find a representative in my area and made an appointment. The woman who came to my home was exceptionally pleasant and professional, but she wore an unattractive, sloppy makeup application and her skin was very dry, which made me nervous (particularly when she told be what great skin care products they had and that she had been with the company for 12 years). I reminded myself that I see plenty of women at the cosmetic counters with poorly applied makeup and I shouldn't let that affect my impression of the products. How the salesperson wears her makeup, good or bad, is not a reflection of the products' quality.

As she unfolded her pink carrying bag and assembled her pinkish display unit filled with pink samples I was surprised to see how totally organized she was. She flipped through a book that explained the products, techniques and company orientation. I was given new demo-sized brushes to use and individualized samples of almost every product (including tiny eye and lip pencils), which was wonderful and impressively sanitary. She explained the order in which to proceed and how to apply the makeup. I did the actual application myself and chose the colors I wanted to try, half following and half ignoring her suggestions. When it was done I looked no better or worse than I had after other makeup applications, which surprised me. I had expected to like none of it, but I ended up liking several of the Mary Kay products.

The major asset to shopping Mary Kay products is the personal service. I felt quite pampered by someone coming to my home to sell me makeup and I was encouraged to test every product before buying a thing. The down side is not knowing who's coming to your door. Every sales representative I met was extremely dedicated to Mary Kay and her products; it felt as if they were talking about a religion, not cosmetics. That kind of intensity is not atypical for cosmetics salespeople, but this kind of devotion to the company head doesn't really exist elsewhere. Another potential problem results from the way the products are marketed: Each salesperson buys her products and samples from the company and sells them directly to the consumer, yet because of cash flow, not all can afford to stock all colors. The tendency then is to show you only what the salesperson has in stock. With all due respect, Mary Kay does have an amazing training program set up for her representatives. The written materials concerning makeup application are remarkable and for the most part completely credible. The Color Logic book, which organizes the makeup colors according to wardrobe, skin and hair colors, is one of the best in the business. The drawback is that not every representative has the talent to recreate what she has learned.

Most of the lipsticks, blushes and foundations have excellent color ranges and good consistency, although the lipsticks do tend toward the greasy side. The colors are conveniently divided into cool, warm and neutral tones. The eyeshadow colors are generally difficult to work with, and almost all of them are too shiny for daytime wear. None of them will reproduce the attractive, conservative, matte makeup look of the women on the Mary Kay brochures. Despite the lack of good eyeshadow colors, Mary Kay is a valid line to look at.

Foundation: Mary Kay has three foundations. Formula 1–Day Radiance, is for very dry skin and the coverage tends to be heavy and thick. Be careful with this one; dry skin doesn't mean you have to wear thick, greasy foundation. Formula 2–Liquid Formula, is for normal to dry skin and is an excellent foundation that gives even coverage. Oil-Free Foundation is for oily skin and provides light coverage. The Oil-Free and Liquid Formula have good consistencies, go on smoothly and have an excellent finish. Day Radiance, which comes in a compact, can go on rather thick and heavy. You have to be careful blending Day Radiance and you want to avoid wearing a powder over it; this foundation already contains talc, and adding more powder will make it look even heavier. I hate to put a damper on what I consider to be a first-rate source of foundation, but Mary Kay's policy is not to sell a foundation to a first-time customer unless she buys the basic skin care products for her skin type. The rationale for this unusual restriction is that the foundation is considered to be part of the skin care routine. They justify this policy by saying they want to monitor allergic reactions and perfect their assessment of your skin type. This sounds good, but all it really means is that you have to buy products that I would otherwise suggest you avoid. So, I'm caught between a rock and a hard place. If I recommend these foundations, I'm also recommending a handful of other products I think aren't worth it. The list of colors I like is presented for your information, but I can't really encourage you to try them if it means you have to buy $50 worth of other products you may not need or want.

Foundation Colors to Try *(all foundations have the same color names)*
Formula 1–Day Radiance ($10)
Misty Ivory: May be too pink for most skin tones.
Creamy Ivory: Great neutral color tone.
Bisque Ivory: Great medium color tone.
Natural Beige: Good color.
Honey Beige: Good color.
Sunlit Beige: Great tan color.
Golden Bronze: May be too orange for some darker skin tones.
Cinnamon Bronze: May be too orange for some darker skin tones.
Classic Bronze: May be too orange for some darker skin tones.
Chestnut Bronze: May be too orange for some darker skin tones.
Deep Bronze: May be too orange for some darker skin tones.

Formula 2–Liquid ($10)
Misty Ivory: May be slightly pink for most skin tones.
Creamy Ivory: May be slightly pink for most skin tones.
Bisque Ivory: Good neutral color tone.
Natural Beige: Good medium color tone.
Honey Beige: Good medium color tone.
Sunlit Beige: Good tan color.
Golden Bronze: Great color for dark skin tones.
Cinnamon Bronze: Great color for dark skin tones.
Classic Bronze: Great color for darker skin tones.
Chestnut Bronze: Great color for darker skin tones.
Deep Bronze: Great color for darker skin tones.

Oil-Free Foundation ($10)
Natural Beige: Good medium skin color.
Bisque Ivory: Great skin color.
Honey Beige: Good medium skin color.
Sunlit Beige: May go on slightly orange, but could be a good
   color for tan or darker skin tones.
Golden Bronze: Great color for darker skin tones.
Cinnamon Bronze: Good color for women of color, though may
   be slightly orange for some skin tones.
Classic Bronze: Good color for African-American women, though
   may be slightly orange for some skin tones.
Chestnut Bronze: Good color for African-American women but
   may turn ashy.
Deep Bronze: Good color for African-American women, but may
   be too orange for some skin tones.

Foundation Colors to Avoid

Formula 1–Day Radiance ($10)
>Light Beige: Too orange for most skin tones.
>Rose Beige: Too orange for most skin tones.

Formula 2–Liquid Formula ($10)
>Light Beige: Too orange.
>Rose Beige: Too orange.

Oil-Free Foundation ($10)
>Misty Ivory: Too pink for most skin tones.
>Creamy Ivory: Too pink for most skin tones.
>Light Beige: Too orange for most skin tones.
>Rose Beige: Too orange.

Concealer: Mary Kay has a Touch On Concealer ($7.50) for covering dark circles under the eye. It is a good product, although the consistency works best on normal to oily skin. Those with dry skin will find it hard to blend, unless they use a moisturizer under the eye area. All the colors — Light, Medium and Dark — are super and definitely worth a try. The representative I talked with encouraged me to put it on my cheek area and nose, but that felt like too much makeup once I put on the foundation.

Finishing Powder: Mary Kay has three shades of Translucent Pressed Powder ($7). All have a soft consistency and go on sheer. The shades are Light, which may be too pink for some skin tones, and Medium and Dark, both of which are great colors and definitely worth a try.

Blush Colors to Try:

Powder Perfect Cheek Color ($7, refill only)
>Azalea: Beautiful soft blush for fair skin tones.
>Wild Rose: May be too bright for some skin tones, but great color.
>Raspberry: Dark skins only.
>Lilac: Nice color.
>Mulberry: May be too brown for some skin tones.
>Cashmere: Good contour color, but may be too orange for some skin tones.
>Apricot: Beautiful coral color.
>Coral: Beautiful color.
>Red Oak: Beautiful color for medium to dark skin tones.

Eyeshadow: I was told by more than one salesperson that the Mary Kay eyeshadows were frostless, which is not the truth. Almost all the colors have too much shine. This is a rather weak link in an otherwise decent product line. The eyeshadows are sold in separate tins that are then placed in a refillable compact. You buy the compact separately and then fill it with the colors of your choice.

Eyeshadow Colors to Try
Powder Perfect Eye Color ($4 per shade, refill only)
Blackest Black: Great color for shading and lining, and no shine.
Periwinkle Bleu: More violet than blue and only slightly shiny, but it is a bright color that is best worn at night.
Classic Navy: Slightly shiny, but a good gray-blue color if you want to wear blue.
Misty Pine: Slightly shiny, but a good gray-green color if you want to wear green.
Exotic Purple: Good for dark skin tones only.
Tuxedo Brown: Slightly shiny, but a good brown color.
Smokey Plum: Slightly shiny, but a good plum color.

Eyeshadow Colors to Avoid
Powder Perfect Eye Color
All of these colors are too shiny: Pink Opal, Pineapple Freeze, Emerald Green (too green), Oyster Shell, Polished Pewter, South Sea (too blue), Spun Silk, Whipped Cocoa, Shimmering Rust (but may be suitable for evening wear), Black Onyx, Oyster Shell (too white), Polished Pewter, Heather Rose.

Lipstick: Mary Kay calls her lipstick Lasting Color Lipstick ($8) but, as is true with almost all lipsticks, how long it really lasts depends on how much you put on, and what you do with your mouth. The consistency is slightly greasy and can feather quickly into the lines around the mouth.

Eye, Lip and Brow Pencils: The Eye Pencil ($6) texture is as good as any I've tried at the department store. The Forest, Slate, Sable and Charcoal are good colors to try. Avoid the Violet and Navy. The Lipliner Pencils ($6) are also great colors and textures. The Brow Pencils ($6) have a slightly slick texture which can make for a shiny brow.

Mascara: Mary Kay's Flawless Mascara ($7) is a decent mascara. It goes on easily and fast, doesn't take a long time to build thickness and doesn't smear, but it is not a great product. Avoid the waterproof variety — it is too difficult to remove. The Conditioning Mascara can smudge, so if you have a problem with mascara smearing by the end of the day, this would not be a good choice.

Specialty Products: Mary Kay sells washable sponges to use when applying your foundation. These are great — some of the best I've seen on the market.

Max Factor

Max Factor was the makeup artist for the rich and famous in the 1920s. He is credited with developing the first mass-produced makeup products that were more than just heavy powder or tints for the cheeks and lips. His task was to find ways to make the men and women in films look exotic, sweet, masterful, wicked, or seductive in a way that was less obvious than on the stage, and this he did with unprecedented flair and creativity. His major creations that have been carried over to the 1990s are Pancake Foundation and Erase, the first foundation and cover stick. I don't recommend that anyone use pancake foundation, but it's nice to recognize the roots of makeup. In terms of the Erase stick, the staple of my youthful days, the texture has become somewhat creamier, there are more colors and it still works well, but the fragrance is too pungent for my personal taste.

Max Factor's lipstick colors are good and each of the four types I tested had an excellent consistency. One of the shades lasted longer on my lips than any other lipstick I tested. Unfortunately, all the lipsticks have an overpowering fragrance. There is an excellent mascara in this line called 2000 Calorie Mascara, and there are some matte eyeshadows that are quite good. Max Factor also has a superior cream-to-powder foundation called Satin Splendor. The colors are great and the texture silky smooth. Unfortunately, the eyeshadows and blushes, for the most part, are too shiny to recommend. To attract a younger, more savvy cosmetics consumer, Max Factor & Co. designed a new product line called Maxi. These products are definitely more contemporary and help bring Max Factor's image up to date.

Foundation: Max Factor still makes a traditional Pancake Foundation ($5.95) and a Panstick Foundation ($5.95). Both are packaged in a sealed plastic wrap that prevents you from viewing the color selections. For that reason alone these are difficult to recommend, and I happen to find the textures of both the pancake and panstick too heavy and thick. Satin Splendor ($7.50), however, is a cream-to-powder foundation that comes in a good selection of colors, has a wonderful consistency, provides sheer but adequate coverage for a natural look, and feels great on the skin. Even without testers you can get fairly close in choosing this one by sight. All the other foundation colors would require testing and none are available.

Concealer: Erase ($3.75) concealer stick is a long-standing Max Factor product. The coverage is good, the consistency creamy without being greasy, and the color choices are excellent. It is not the best on dry skin, however, unless you put on a moisturizer first. Unfortunately, it also has an intense fragrance that prevents me from recommending it wholeheartedly. Erase is the only undereye concealer that comes in a white shade, which works best for correcting dark circles under the eye. If you can take the fragrance, it's worth checking out. There is also a waterproof Erase stick that I don't recommend; you have to remove it with an oil-based cleanser that usually needs to be wiped off instead of rinsed.

Finishing Powder: Max Factor makes a Creme Puff Pressed Powder ($5.75) that is packaged in such a way that the powder puff blocks the view of the color. Therefore, I can't recommend it.

Blush Colors to Try
Satin Blush ($2.95)
> All of these colors are soft and beautiful: Pinkamelon, Porcelain Peach, Tiger Lily, Mulled Wine, Tender Rouge, Subtle Amber (a good contour color), Pink Velvet, Mauve Rose and Tea Rose.

Blush Colors to Avoid
Satin Blush ($2.95)
> All of these are too shiny: Sangria, Crystal Sherry, Freshwater Pink, Topaz, Desert Pink, Wild Rose, Shimmering Lilac and Midnight Rose.

New Definition Perfecting Blush ($6.95)
The colors are all fine, but the texture of this cream-to-powder blush is somewhat grainy and not one I would recommend.
Maxi-Glow ($2.75)
This is a very lightweight cream blush, that has a beautiful consistency for cream blush. All of the colors are lovely, but the color just doesn't last: Apricoral, Pinkberry, Bittersweet Pink and Ginger Peach.

Eyeshadow Colors to Try
Picture Perfect Eyeshadows ($2.95)
All of these are excellent colors: Grey Flannel, Cafe au Lait, Sweet Lilac, Country Pink (good color for darker skin tones).
Maxi Color-to-Go ($1.50)
Stormy Weather: Can be a good gray blue for some skin tones. Abstract Pink: Good pink for darker skin tones.

Eyeshadow Colors to Avoid
Picture Perfect Eyeshadows ($2.95)
All of these colors are too shiny: Creme de Menthe (too green) Tapestry Mauve, Perfect Perle, True Blue (no shine, but too blue) Sable, Pink Bouquet, Jade, Champagne, Sky Blue, Blue Lace, Soft Suede, Black Velvet, Brilliant Blue, Soft Teal, Blue Ice and Karat.
Maxi Colors-to-Go ($1.50)
All of these colors are too shiny: Goldilocks, Light-as-a-Feather, Medium Rare, Mint Julip, Terrific Teal, Aqua Marine (too blue-green), Blackout, China Sea, Blue Angle (too blue), Paper Moon (can be too white for most skin tones), Blue Lagoon (too blue) and Faded Jeans (too blue).
Shadow Blocks ($3.95)
All of the colors are too shiny. It's a shame, because the concept of stamping each color with a bold letter that represents where you apply the color is clever; "A" for accent color, "B" for base color and "C" for contour color, to help you with your application.

Lipstick: Except for the intense fragrance, I loved the Max Factor selection of lipsticks: Moisture Rich Lipstick ($4.75), New Definition ($4.95), Lasting Color Lipstick ($4.75) and — my favorite — Maxi's Soft Lustre Long Lasting Lipstick ($2.65). They were all extremely creamy and the color really lasted. Maxi's Not Quite Lipstick ($2.65) is more of a gloss that a lipstick. Maxi's Soft Lustre Lipstick has to be one of the best lipstick buys on the market. If you can take the somewhat sweet odor that all these lipsticks have, they're great.

Lip, Eye and Brow Pencils: Max Factor has a Brush & Brow ($5.25) powder that colors in the eyebrow with a hard brush. The color selection is excellent: Smokey Grey, Soft Black, Natural Brown, Midnight Brown and Ash Blond. The powder works beautifully, but the firm brush is hard on the brow. It would be better to use these colors with a soft brush. There is a Maxi Color Kohl Liner ($2.10) that has a pencil at one end and a sponge tip at the other for blending. The darker shades like Black and Hot Fudge are good, but stay away from the brighter shades which are too shiny. Max Factor's Featherblend Kohliners ($4.95) are an excellent assortment of eye pencils; one end is a brush, which blends better than the more typical sponge-tips that come with these two-in-one type pencils. Quick Draw Magic Eyeliner Pen ($4.95) is a felt-tip liquid eyeliner that can make eye look obviously lined. There is also a Lip Definer ($4.95) pencil that is wonderful; one end is a lipstick brush which can be convenient. Maxi's Lip Contouring Pencil ($2.65) comes in a poor selection of colors and has a fairly greasy texture. Max Factor makes a lip cream called Lip Renew ($5) that comes in a tube and is supposed to prevent lipstick from bleeding. It did not work as well as I would have liked and I do not prefer this type of anti-feathering product because it makes reapplication difficult.

Mascara: The Max Factor line has one of the better mascaras on the market. 2000 Calorie Mascara ($4.95) goes on easily, doesn't smear, and makes lashes thick and long. It tends to flake if you overbuild the lashes. Don't overdo and it should last the whole day. Maxi-Lash ($2.50) doesn't work nearly as well as the 2000 Calorie Mascara or many others on the market. Several coats left my lashes short and relatively undefined. They also have a No-Coat Mascara. At ($4.95) it's expensive for a clear gel that leaves the lashes in pretty much the same shape as before you used it. This would do the trick for those who want just a tinge of extra length over already dark eyelashes.

Maybelline

I have a vivid memory of making my first makeup purchases from Maybelline. I can see the colors of blue, brown and white vividly through the clear plastic wrapper. I can also remember the pride I felt as I took out my own money and paid for my first steps toward maturity. Maybelline and I go back a long way, but I hadn't purchased Maybelline products for years until I started the research for this book. I found the blue cardboard packaging to be ever so familiar, but this time the selections seemed comparatively extensive. (Or maybe it's just that now I look for more than just blue, brown and white eyeshadows.)

In spite of my fond memories of Maybelline, I can only recommend a handful of interesting products. Some of the blush colors are worth checking into, there is a small selection of beautiful matte eyeshadows, and there is also a unique variety of eyelining pencils to consider. Maybelline does make one of my favorite inexpensive mascaras — Great Lash Mascara — but that's about it. The foundation colors are, for the most part, too pink or peach to recommend. Most of the eyeshadows and lipsticks are fabulous colors, but extremely shiny. The pencils and lipsticks are packaged in containers that disguise the colors. And the translucent powders, although they have an excellent texture and decent color, are also packaged so that you can't see the color clearly. Maybelline has a line of oil-free products for the teenage market called Shine Free. They are advertised as being non-acnegenic or non-comedogenic. Claims like these are always enticing but don't usually pan out. I tried their Shine Free Liquid Makeup and developed a few blemishes immediately afterwards.

Foundation: There are no foundation testers in this line so no recommendations can be made. Maybelline has six types of foundations: Long-Wearing Makeup, Sheer Essential, Moisture Whip, Shine-Free, and Ultra-Performance. Almost all of the foundations I purchased in each of these categories were all too pink or peach except for Sheer Essential.

Concealer: Cover Stick Waterproof Concealer ($3.35) comes in four reliable shades and has a soft creamy consistency, but too much fragrance. Shine Free Cover Stick ($3.50) comes in Light and Medium. Both colors and texture are good, and it doesn't crease. There is also a basic Cover Stick that comes in three reliable shades, but this one tends to crease.

Finishing Powder: Translucent Pressed Powder ($4) contains talc and mineral oil, and the Satin Complexion Pressed Powder ($4) contains talc and no oil. Both of these are ok and the colors are good, but the powder has a tendency to go on chalky.

Blush: Maybelline has a wide range of blush colors that are worth trying. The only thing to be aware of is that many of these shades go on very soft and sheer no matter how much of the color you apply. If you are looking for vivid colors this is not the line to consider.

Blush Colors to Try
Brush/Blush I, II, III ($4)

All are excellent colors: Misty Pink, Fresh Peach, Gentle Rose, Seashell Pink, Pink Carnation, Raspberry Whisper, Sweetheart Rose, Barely Pink, Primrose, Pink Mist, Parfait Pink Trio, Plumberry Collection, Misty Pink/Pink Peony, Pink Chiffon/Soft Heather, Terracotta Rose (slightly shiny), Pretty in Peach (slightly shiny) and Pink Blush (slightly shiny).

Eyeshadow: Maybelline has several types of eyeshadow. The ones to absolutely avoid are the Cream-On Eyeshadow ($3.70) — the colors are too shiny, bright, hard to blend and limited. Color Wand ($4.50) is a pencil that dispenses eyeshadow onto a sponge-tip applicator; most of the colors are too shiny. The same is true for Color Wand II ($5.90), half real pencil and the other half an eyeshadow. The Color Wand is an interesting idea, but the eye-pencil part is too fat to maintain a good point and the eyeshadow colors are too shiny.

Eyeshadow Colors to Try
Singles, Duos, Trios and Quads: ($1.95–$4.50)

All of these colors are beautiful and matte: Sunset Colors, Royal Velvet, Ruby Satin (for darker skin tones), Barely Pink, Shy Violet, Lilac Velvet, Butter-Me-Up, Brown Sugar (one color is shiny, but otherwise it's great), Grey Suede, Champagne Brunch, Seashell Pink, The Watercolors, The Suedes and Earthy Taupe.

Eyeshadow Colors to Avoid
Singles, Duos, Trios and Quads ($1.95–$4.50)

All of these colors are too shiny: Pick-a-Plum, Newport Blue, I Got

The Blues, Blue Notes, Box of Chocolates, Berry Nice, Over the Rainbow, Autumn Leaves, Patelle Palette, Quick Silver Blues, Ice Blue, Blue Bell, Stormy Blue, Blue Blazes, Marine Green, Aquarius, Soft Plum Frosts, Misty Blue Frosts, Seashore Frosts, Ideal Blues, Misty Mint and Soft White (too white for most skin tones). Warning: All of the Shine-Free eyeshadows are irridescent. Did they think we wouldn't notice?

Lipstick: Maybelline's Long-Wearing Lipstick ($3.75) has a very slippery, creamy texture and goes on quite soft. Moisture Whip ($3.75) has a slightly drier texture than the Long-Wearing Lipstick, but only slightly. And Slim Lipstick ($4.75) is more gloss than lipstick and many of the shades are frosted. I don't dislike the Maybelline lipsticks, but they are a bit too greasy for everyday wear and the color selection is limited. But for a more sheer look, Long-Wearing Lipstick and Moisture Whip Lipstick are excellent.

Lip, Eye and Brow Pencils: Maybelline has five types of pencil for lining the eye. Perfect Pen Eyeliner and Lineworks ($5.25) are both felt-tip liquid liners that are almost identical. Both dry to a somewhat shiny, slick finish and create a very obvious "lined" look. Expert Eyes ($3.75) is an automatic pencil with a sponge tip at one end. On top of the pencil there is a device that allows you to sharpen the pencil to an even finer point. Turning Point Eyeliner ($4.75) is an automatic pencil that turns out a point that is really too thick to use reliably as an eyeliner. Performing Colors ($3.50) is a traditional eye pencil that comes in a small assortment of colors. For all the variety, the only product worth investigating is the Expert Eyes eyelining pencil. You won't be able to see the color you're buying, but if you're looking for black or brown, this is an excellent product. For the lips, Maybelline's Precision Lip Liner ($4) is great, but the color selection is limited.

Mascara: Maybelline makes one of my favorite mascaras, Great Lash Mascara ($3.75). It goes on easily, builds good length and doesn't smear. Not bad for the money. There are several other mascaras in this line, but the only other one I really liked was No Problem Mascara ($3.95). The others were mediocre — I found none to be as good as the Great Lash or No Problem. Their new mascara, Perfectly Natural ($3.25) is ok, but it doesn't build up much thickness.

Origins

Estee Lauder starts off the 1990s with a new cosmetics line called Origins and what a concept it is. The quote from one of the brochures sums it up quite nicely: "Origins marries the forces of nature with the vigor of modern science to make provocative differences in the way you experience cosmetics." To put it in my own words: "Origins utilizes all the current fads on the market to create one of the most distinct makeup and skin care collections around." The brochures, like most of the packaging, are all made of recycled paper. The ad copy is loaded with names of exotic-sounding botanicals, herbs and oils. References to Egyptian and Roman know-how are frequent. If you're looking for the allure of "natural" products, none comes as close as Origins to living up to that claim. Modern science plays a part in the technical-sounding promotions that describe theories about skin care and makeup application. It's going to be hard to ignore this line in the 90s. They even sell sensory therapy oils and gels that are "thousands of years old." Of course, the oils and gels aren't that old, but the idea is to convince you that whoever was around thousands of years ago must have used these concoctions, and that must be good.

I was very impressed with the color presentation at the Origins counter. The lipsticks, eyeshadows, blushes and lip pencils are divided into three color groupings: Peach to Rust, Beige to Tan, and Ivory to Pink. All of the colors have minimal or no shine and most of the colors are soft and muted and therefore extremely easy to use. The textures are wonderful and the application is almost flawless. Although I like the eyeshadows, be aware that there is some amount of shine present; many of the salespeople I talked to insisted that the colors were all matte and they are not. There is also a problem with the amount of flower extract used in many of the Origins products. If you have any hayfever-type allergies, these are going to cause you problems. "Natural" ingredients are not automatically the best for all skin types.

Foundation: There are only two foundation types, which is refreshing when you consider that almost every other cosmetics line has four or five types from which to choose. Each of the foundations has a good, light consistency. Unfortunately, the Moisture Makeup comes in an extremely poor assortment of colors and contains talc and kaolin, which are terrible for dry skin. For those reasons, I mostly recommend the Matte Makeup.

Foundation Colors to Try

Moisture Makeup ($16)
   Birch: Excellent color.
Matte Makeup ($16)
   All of these colors are excellent: Blossom, Shell, Flax, Linen and
   Chestnut.

Foundation Colors to Avoid

Moisture Makeup ($16)
   All of these colors are either too orange or pink: Ginger, Sugar
   Cane, Biscuit, Vanilla, Coffee, Cocoa (too ashy-green), Honey and
   Sand (very orange).
Matte Makeup ($16)
   Allspice: Too ashy-green for most skin tones.
   Maple: Can turn peach on most skin tones.
   Wheat: Too orange.

Finishing Powder: Origins Translucent Powder ($17.50) are all mica-
and talc-based. They are soft and sheer, although it's hard to imagine
who would use some of these colors. Nature's Cream, Nature's Almond
and Nature's Copper are good colors; Nature's Peach is too peach,
Nature's Rose is too pink and Alabaster is pure white.

Concealer: Origins concealer ($10) comes in two shades. Light is an
excellent shade, but Medium can be too peach for most skin tones. This
is a fine concealer inspite of the limited color selection.

Blush Colors to Try ($15)

   All the blush colors are superb and unquestionably worth a try:
   Nutmeg, Persimmon, Nectar, Orchid, Laurel, Hyacinth, Claret,
   Tulip, Brick and Dusk.

Eyeshadow: Origins has a superb array of matte eyeshadows. Although
I dislike almost all shades of bright blue and green eyeshadows in
general, I feel that almost all the eyeshadow colors in this line are
worth a try. Even the blues are some of the nicest blues on the market.
Warning: Not all these colors are matte; a very few do have a small
amount of shine.

Eyeshadow Colors to Try
Singles ($12.50)

All of these colors are splendid: Quince, Seashell, Cayenne, Cinnamon, Primrose, Cabernet, Daphne, Sherry, Rosebud, Driftwood, Raisin, Winter Bloom, Umber, Snow (may be too white for most skin tones), Mocha, Blue Sage (may be too blue for most skin tones), Tourmaline (may be too blue for most skin tones), Malachite (may be too green for most skin tones), Olive, Kiwi (may be too green for most skin tones), Maize, Pineapple, Lapis, Wisteria, Iris, Heather, Amethyst, Fog (superb shade of gray), Slate and Onyx.

Lipstick: I wish I could say I like Origin's lipsticks ($10), because the color choices are simply stunning. But the texture is too glossy and the color won't survive to the mid-morning break. If you have a problem with lipstick bleeding into the lines around your mouth, you'll feel this lipstick traveling the second you put it on.

Eye, Brow and Lip Pencils: The Eye and Lip Pencils ($9) come in great colors, though the selection is limited. The Brow Pencil ($9), like all brow pencils, has a slightly slick texture and are not recommended unless you are a wizard at penciling brows that don't look fake.

Mascara: Origins makes only one product that I would call somewhat gimmicky: Underwear for Lashes. It is an undercoating for the lashes that you apply before the mascara. The claim is that it helps the lashes grab more mascara. A good mascara should suffice, so this is an unnecessary layer on fragile lashes.

Prescriptives

Prescriptives is an extension, or cousin, of Estee Lauder, but that is about all they have in common. Many of the reservations I have about the makeup products in the Estee Lauder line are eliminated when I consider many of Prescriptives' products. Almost all their colors — blush, eyeshadows, lipstick, pencils and powders — are matte with no shine whatsoever. Now that's a find! The major problem is that selecting a product is somewhat complicated, at least from a consumer's point of view. The counter personnel I interviewed had a wide variety of training, and this line requires training — you're better off talking to someone who has been with the line for a while. Actually that's true for almost all lines, but more so with this one.

The counter displays are incredibly well organized and the color selections, for the most part, are terrific. All the shades are divided into four color groups: yellow/orange, red, red/orange, and blue/red. It is the job of the salesperson to color-type your skin, and to indicate what foundations and principal color group you should be wearing. The hitch is, once you know what your principal color group is, you are told that you can wear certain colors in all the other groups for a more natural, dramatic or intensified look. Not a concept that everyone would agree with, particularly me, but a great theory for selling more products. No matter how the woman tried to convince me that I would look great in yellow/orange colors for my natural look, there is no way I felt comfortable in those shades. In spite of this sales tenet, I like their color selections and find many of their products to be quite good. And almost all of Prescriptives products are fragrance-free.

Foundation: Prescriptives has five types of foundation made for a variety of skin types — a total of 67 shades altogether. Makeup 1 is an excellent light foundation designed for normal to dry skin; Makeup 2 is for dry skin and has a somewhat heavier coverage than Makeup 1. 100% Oil-Free Liquid Makeup is a very good oil-free foundation designed for oily to combination skin that provides a sheer light coverage. Oil-Free Foundation is half glycerin and water which floats at the top of the jar, while the other half, talc, sits on the bottom until you shake it (and you have to shake it vigorously to mix it thoroughly). This is a tricky product to use and I don't recommend it. Furthermore, in concentrated amounts, glycerin can cause allergic reactions. Custom Blend is prepared for you personally and assumes that the salesperson can match your skin tone better by mixing and matching than by selling you the ready-made shades they have. I did not review the custom blend foundation. Custom blend sounds like a good idea, but it relies too much on the expertise of the individual salesperson.

A specific foundation shade is chosen for you from the existing foundation colors by a process they call "color printing." Four of the potential foundation color groups are drawn in a line on your cheek with the Makeup 1 foundation and then allowed to dry. One will seem to disappear into your skin and that is considered the foundation color group that is best for you. Within the color group chosen for you, there is a range of shades from light to dark. I found this to be one of the more reliable ways to test foundation, except that the final selection can vary from salesperson to salesperson. Some of the foundation colors that are "accepted" by your skin may still look too pink or orange in the sunlight, and there is still the question of proper intensity. Regardless of how scientific color printing sounds, be sure to check the foundation in the daylight to assure true compatibility.

Foundation Colors to Try

Oil-Free Liquid ($28.50)

Yellow-Orange Suntan: Beautiful color for darker skin tones.

Yellow Orange Tuscan Beige: Beautiful color for tan to medium skin tones.

Yellow-Orange Rich Gold: Beautiful medium to tan shade.

Yellow-Orange True Bisque: Great neutral shade.

Yellow-Orange Fresh Ivory: This has no yellow in it, and it may turn slightly pink on some skin tones.

Blue-Red Pure Porcelain: Good color for deeper skin tones, but may turn slightly pink.

Blue-Red Rose Silk: Good color for deeper skin tones, but may turn slightly pink.

Red-Orange Copper Beige: Great medium shade.

Red-Orange Quiet Beige: Great medium shade.

Makeup 1 ($28.50)

Red-Orange Verona Beige: Great color choice.

Red-Orange Fresh Peach: nothing peach about this color, great color choice.

Yellow-Orange Pale Gold: Great natural beige tone.

Yellow-Orange Bisque: Great natural beige tone.

Yellow-Orange Ivory Silk: Great natural beige tone.

Yellow-Orange Pale Cream: Excellent shade for fair skin tones.

Yellow-Orange Fresh Cream: Great neutral shade for fair skin tones.

Yellow-Orange Burnished Gold: Excellent color for medium skin tones.

Blue-Red Rosewood: Good color for darker skin tones.

Blue-Red Victorian Porcelain: Good color for medium to darker skin tones.

Red-Orange Cyprus Umber: Good bronze color.

Red-Orange Mosaic Gold: Good tan color, but can turn orange on some skin tones.

Red-Orange Amber Beige: Good medium color, but can turn peach on some skin tones.

Red-Orange Warm Peach: Great color for fair to medium skin tones.

Makeup 2 ($28.50)

Red-Orange Sunny Peach: Good medium to tan color, but can turn peach on some skin tones.

Red-Orange Amber: Good tan color but may turn peach.

Yellow-Orange Tan: Great color for darker skin tones.

Yellow-Orange Perfect Bisque: Good color for fair to medium skin tones.

Yellow-Orange Rich Cream: Great color for fair skin tones.

Yellow-Orange Creamy Gold: Great neutral color.

Yellow-Orange Soft Ivory: Great neutral color.

Blue-Red Fresh Camellia: Good for fair skin tones, but may turn pink.

Blue-Red English Porcelain: Good for fair to medium skin tones, but may turn pink.

Foundation Colors to Avoid

Oil-Free Liquid ($28.50)

Yellow-Orange Soft Gold: May be slightly peach for most skin tones.

Blue-Red Rose Earth: May turn peach.

Blue-Red Tea Rose: May turn pink on some skin tones.

Blue-Red Pale Alabaster: Too pink for most skin tones.

Red-Orange Pure Gold: Too peach for most skin tones.

Red-Orange Roman Peach: Good color, but may turn peach on some skin tones.

Red-Orange Natural Peach: May be too pink for most skin tones.

Makeup 1 ($28.50)

All of these shades are all too peachy-pink; Blue-Red Porcelain, Blue-Red Alabaster, Blue-Red Camellia, Blue-Red Rose Porcelain, Red Pale Blush and Red Warm Blush.

Makeup 2 ($28.50)

Red-Orange Classic Beige: Ok color, but can be too peach.

Red-Orange Pure Peach: The name is accurate, this is too peach for most skin tones.

Blue-Red Almond: Can turn rose on most skin tones.

Blue-Red Rose Cameo: Can turn rose on most skin tones.

Blue-Red Cool Alabaster: Extremely pink, almost lavender.
Red Outdoor Blush — Extremely peach.

Concealer: Prescriptives has 11 shades of concealer called Camouflage Cream ($12.50). Most of the colors are for those with medium skin tones; there are only one or two colors for fair to medium skin tones, but these colors are great. The consistency is somewhat creamy when it goes on, slightly dry when blended and doesn't crease. It is an excellent product, but there are cheaper concealers that are just as good in other less expensive lines.

Concealer Colors to Try

Yellow-Orange Light: Great color for medium skin tones.
Yellow-Orange Medium: Great color for medium to dark skin tones.
Yellow-Orange Dark: Great color for darker skin tones.
Red-Orange Light: Good color.
Red-Orange Medium: Beautiful color.
Red-Orange Dark: Beautiful color.
Blue-Red Light: Great color for fair skin tones.
Red-Orange Extra Dark: Excellent color for women of color.

Concealer Colors to Avoid

Red Light: Too pink.
Blue-Red Medium: Too peach.
Blue-Red Dark: Too peach.

Finishing Powder: The Better Pressed Powder ($22.50) is talc-based and contains mineral oil. It is available in a great selection of colors. The loose powder comes in two types; Oil Control ($20) contain talc, zinc and clay; and Moisture Rich ($20) contains talc, mineral and lanolin oil. All have a silky soft texture.

Blush: All the blush colors ($18.50) are worth trying. These are beautiful shades with no visible shine, although some of the colors tend to go on quite sheer. The browner tones—Sandalwood, Cherrywood, Tulipwood and Rosewood — are superb contour colors.

Eyeshadow Colors to Try
Singles, Duos and Quads ($16/$30/$30)

A superior collection beautiful matte colors: Red Orange, Red, Blue Red, Yellow Orange, Brown Ink, Wheat (slightly shiny) Walnut, Saffron (strange shade of green-yellow), Sandstone, Bottle Green (accent color only), Ocean (if you have to wear blue, this is the shade to try), Admiral (evening wear), Slate (more blue than gray; be careful), Fog (exquisite shade of soft gray), Rose Powder, Flesh, Peach Dust, Pongee, Heliotrope, Coal, Elephant and Violet.

Eyeshadow Colors to Avoid
Singles Only ($16)

All these colors are too shiny: Mustard, Chrome Green (too lime green for most skin tones), Ultramarine (too blue), Rose Quartz, Pink Satin, Venetian Gold and Chutney.

Lipstick: Prescriptives has Classic ($12.50) and Demi-Matte ($14) lipsticks. The Classic is by far the preferred choice with its nice array of colors and good consistency. The Demi-Matte colors are dark and the texture is dry. These shades change every season, so the chances of finding a certain selection again are slim. The line offers a gloss, but there is no reason to spend this much money on a gloss.

Eye, Brow and Lip Pencils: Prescriptives has a huge selection of lip and eye pencil ($12) colors that have a great texture but are not unusual as far as pencils go. The eye pencils come in good colors, but they are crayon-like and go on too greasy.

Mascara: Prescriptives has an excellent mascara ($12). There is only one mascara in this line, a simplification I much appreciated; most other lines have at least four mascaras with minor differences.

Revlon (Department Store)

I wanted to like Revlon's department store products more than I did. A reasonably priced department-store brand of cosmetics could be the best of both worlds: department store service and drugstore prices. At Revlon's counter you definitely get the service. Almost all the salespeople I talked to were helpful. The displays on the counter were easily accessible and I was encouraged to try samples on my own. For those who like to use their own personal expertise as opposed to the salesperson's, this is always a plus. The down side is that many of the foundation colors are too orange or pink, and the eyeshadows are too shiny, even though they have a great silky texture. This line is most appropriate for women of color or women with dark skin tones, because the shades are so strong. The lipsticks were also a disappointment. The texture was very greasy, and the lipstick squashed when placed on the lips with very little pressure. If you want a glossy look, these lipsticks will be fine; if you have a problem with lipsticks bleeding into the lines around your mouth, this is not the product for you. The up side is that the blush colors are beautiful and the textures soft and silky, and there are a handful of new matte eyeshadows that are fabulous and worth checking out.

Foundation: Revlon's two foundation types have good textures, but also their problems. Only the Photofinish Makeup for oily skin is noteworthy; it is a traditional liquid foundation that dries to a powder. The problem is getting it to go on evenly if you don't use a sponge (although that's true for any foundation type, it is even more true for this one). Once the liquid dries, it is hard to smooth out the powder residue. The Colorlift Makeup for normal to dry skin is a decent product, but the color choice is poor, which makes it difficult to recommend. The foundations in this line are primarily for women with darker skin tones.

Foundation Colors to Try

Colorlift Makeup ($12.50)
>   Fawn Beige: Good color for darker skin tones.
>   Sahara Sands: Worth a try, but may be slightly pink for some skin tones.
>   Wheat: Great color, but may turn yellow on some skin tones.
>   Toasted Almond: Great color for tan or darker skin tones.

Photofinish Makeup ($11.50)
>   Ivory Cream: Good color for fair skin tones.
>   Pink Buff: Ignore the "pink" name; the color is good for fair skin tones.
>   Sandy Beige: Good color for tan skin tones.
>   Driftwood Beige: Good for tan or darker tones.
>   Honey Wheat: Good color for tan or darker skin tones.

Foundation Colors to Avoid

Colorlift Makeup ($12.50)

> Cool Ivory: May be too pink for most fair skin tones.
> Pink Bisque: Too pink for most skin tones.
> Earth Rose: Too orange.
> Peach Nectar: Too orange.
> Island Tan: May be too orange for most darker skin tones.

Photofinish Makeup ($11.50)

> Tawny Rose — too orange
> Golden Peach — may turn orange
> Caribbean Tan — too orange

Concealer: Revlon has something called Eye Makeup Prepstick ($9) which comes in a dual-purpose tube that has liquid concealer at one end and eyeshadow base at the other end. Because I don't recommend using an extra eyeshadow base, this product is not high on my list. The concealer, however, happens to be excellent; it doesn't crease, but because of its dry consistency, it is best for those with normal to oily skin. The concealer comes in three shades: Light, which is too pinkish-orange; Medium and Dark are both ok for darker skin tones only. The eyeshadow base that accompanies all the concealers is pink, a poor color choice for the lid and for most skin tones in general. A foundation and powder would create the same finish.

Finishing Powder: Revlon's Silkscreen Powder ($10) has a soft consistency and goes on rather sheer, but the color choice is poor. The Light is too pink for most skin tones; Medium and Dark are good for medium and tan skin tones only.

Blush Colors to Try

Color Cling Blush ($10)

> All these colors are gorgeous: Neutral Ivory, Neutral Fawn, Neutral Nude, Neutral Pewter, Neutral Mimosa, Neutral Cayenne, Neutral Umber (excellent contour color), Neutral Tan (excellent contour color), Bronzetta (very shiny, evening wear only), Shell Pink (beautiful; pale pink; fair skin tones only), Nectarina, Plummery, Begonia (intense pink, best for darker skin tones), Winery (good plum color for darker skin tones) and Poppy.

Eyeshadow Colors to Try

Color Cling Eyeshadows ($9)

Mimosa: Beautiful color, very little shine.

Opalesque: For evening wear only, can be a tricky color to use.

Beachrose: Beautiful color, for dark skin tones only.

Cayenne: Great brown-rose tone, good for lining and shading.

Petalpink: No shine in this color, but it may be too white for most skin tones.

Lilacreme: Soft light lilac, but may be too white for most skin tones.

Flamingo: Intense pink; for darker skin tones only.

Boysenberry: Opalescent violet; for evening wear only.

Eyeshadow Colors to Avoid

Color Cling Eyeshadows ($9)

Copperlite: Very shiny; for evening wear only.

Driftwood: Too shiny.

Olivine: Too shiny.

Sasparilla: Very shiny, for evening wear only.

Turquoise: Very, very blue.

Charcoalite: Looks more blue than gray.

Blue Note: Speaks for itself.

Mediterranean Blue: Speaks for itself.

Lipstick: Revlon's "Self-Renewing" ($9) formula is very greasy and bleeds almost immediately after you apply it. The shiny look the colors impart is not my favorite. If you like this kind of lipstick, the color selection is fine; otherwise I don't recommend it.

Revlon (Drugstore)

When I started reviewing drugstore lines, I began with Revlon. I was surprised at how much I liked the experience. If nothing else, it was a kick to take home one of almost everything and have a bill that was literally a fraction of the cost of five or six products from the department store. This is a huge product line with many choices and color options, not to mention some of the most gimmicky specialty items I've seen in any cosmetics line. For example, they have a blusher called Air Blush ($7.95): You pump the back of the brush handle to release the powder into the brush. I found it messy to use and not worth the price, but it was definitely a unique concept.

Revlon makes an assortment of foundations, most of which are fairly orange and peach, but recently they came out with a product called Springwater Makeup that is oil-free and most of the colors are refreshingly neutral. There are a handful of matte eyeshadows in this collection, that are great choices and almost embarrassingly inexpensive. The lipsticks are for the most part wonderful; I particularly like the creamy texture of Moondrops Super Lustrous Creme, and the colors are excellent. The assortment of eyelining options is also extensive and most of the colors, particularly those that aren't bright and shiny, are excellent. The lipliners, too, are very good. One word of caution: Some of the lip and eye liners are waterproof, and I don't like recommending them because they can only be removed with an oil-based cleanser.

Foundation: Revlon has three types of foundation in its drugstore line: New Complexion Makeup for Normal to Dry, New Complexion Makeup for Normal to Oily, and Touch & Glow Makeup. Almost every shade is either too pink, orange, peach or rose. I can't recommend any of them. Exceptions are Revlon's Powder Creme Makeup base, which is a good product with a smooth texture and easy application, and Springwater Oil-Free Makeup ($7.95) which is a superior foundation in mostly neutral shades of beige or tan. What a relief! Thank you, Revlon. It's about time. Now include tester units in your display, as does L'Oreal, so that women can make intelligent decisions about the foundation they buy.

Foundation Colors to Try
Powder Creme Makeup ($6.95)

Fresh Beige: May be slightly pink for some skin tones.

Delicate Ivory: Good color for very fair skin tones.

Tender Peach: Good color but may be turn rose on some skin tones.

Warm Beige: Good color for medium skin tones.

Healthy Tan: Good for dark skin tones only, can turn rose on some skin tones.

Concealer: Revlon's New Complexion Concealer ($6.50) comes in three shades: Light, Medium and Deep. This is a lightweight concealer that leaves a sheer residue that covers beautifully. This is one of the better concealers I tested. It is definitely worth looking into. This line also has a Vanishing Stick ($5.50) that comes in colors that are very yellow and peach; it is also highly fragranced and goes on rather thick. And finally, Wear & Care Eyeshadow Base ($5.25) is similar (if not identical) to the eyeshadow base Revlon sells at the department store. It is not a necessary element; I find it makes no difference in how the makeup lasts during the day.

Finishing Powder: Revlon has a good selection of pressed powders. They are all talc-based and go on soft. The problem is the color selection; many of these shades are a bit too peach or pink for most skin tones.

Finishing Powder Colors to Try
Love Pat Pressed Powder ($5.75)
> Soft Beige: Good color for medium skin tones.
> Translucent Natural: May turn pink on some fair skin tones.
> Translucent No. 2: Can be slightly pink for some skin tones.
Springwater Powder Oil-Free ($7.95)
> Light: Good color choice.
> Medium: Good color color.
> Dark: Good color choice.

Finishing Powder Colors to Avoid
Love Pat Pressed Powder ($5.75)
> All these colors are too peach for most skin tones: Cream Beige, Cream Ivory, Suntan, Rachel, Misty Rose, and Translucent No. 1 (too pink for most skin tones).

Blush: Revlon has an interesting assortment of blushes that range from ultra-frost, which is too intense for daytime, to soft, exceptional colors that are great any time. My favorite is Powder Creme Blush, a superb product with a silky texture that glides on smooth and evenly. It would be hard to make your cheeks look overdone with this blusher.

Blush Colors to Try
Glamorous Blush-On ($6.95)
> Revlon Red: Good color for darker skin tones only.
> Mauve: Good color for darker skin tones only.
> Wine: Good soft plum color.

Sandalwood Beige: Great contour color.

Neutral Umber: Excellent contour color.

Neutral Tan: Excellent contour color.

Bronzetta: Excellent contour color.

Powder Creme Blush ($6.25)

All of these colors are great: Amberfrost, Pink, Mauvefrost, Primrose and Plum.

Sheer Face Color ($5.25)

All of these colors are excellent: Sheer Tawny (great contour color), Sheer Rose, Sheer Peach and Sheer Pink.

Blush Colors to Avoid

Pure Radiance ($7.15)

Original Sun Glow: This color is supposed to be used as a bronzer. It is not a great idea to change the color of the skin; no matter how good the color is, you always end up with a color at the jaw or on your collar.

Soft Lustre Blush ($6.95)

All of these colors are too shiny: Fresh Peach, Sunrise Pink, Rose Lustre, Irrepressible Rose and Honey Brown Lustre.

Eyeshadow: Revlon has a superior selection of matte eyeshadows that I feel comfortable recommending to anyone who wants a soft natural-looking eye design. You can buy a compact to hold the pop-in tins that you buy separately from the rack, but the pop-in tins can easily be used without the compact. Be careful — not all the colors are matte, and most have quite a bit of shine. Revlon offers a Powder Pencil, but all the colors are too shiny and I don't recommend eyeshadows that cannot be blended easily with a brush.

Eyeshadow Colors to Try

Singles and Duos ($2.50)

All of these are excellent colors: Beaches, Dawn, Twilight (fair skin tones), Desert, Slated Grey, Granite, Cedar, Rose Briar (darker skin tones only), Currantine (darker skin tones) Bluestone (if you have to wear blue, this will do), Not Quite White, Bali Brown (good liner or accent color), Ranch Mink (good liner or accent color), Peach Whisper, Slightly Pink (may be too white for some skin tones) and Lilac Lucense (intense lilac color, darker skin tones).

Overtime Shadows ($4.95)

All of these colors are beautiful: Nudes, Mauvestones, Lilacs and Naturals.

Eyeshadow Colors to Avoid

Singles and Duos ($2.50)

All of these colors are too shiny: Dusty Pink Frost, Cameo Blush, Superfrost Pink, Mauve Gold, Baby Blue, China Blue Frost (speaks for itself), Silverlace, Mint Julip, Superfrost Beige, Peach Blast, Burnished Khaki, Ipanema Gold, Taupestar, Sheer Sky, Clear Seas (too blue), Gauze Grey (too blue), Aquarium (no shine, but too blue). Paradise Matte, Lilac Matte and Smokies Matte have no shine, but each contains two or more blues, and who needs more blue eyeshadows?

Overtime Shadows ($4.95)

All of these colors are too shiny: Smokies (too blue), Foliage, Paradise (too blue) and Aquatines (too green).

Lipstick: Revlon makes three types of lipstick which are all excellent. Super Lustrous Creme ($5.25), Moon Drop Moisture Creme ($5.25) and Moon Drop Luminesque ($5.25). All are wonderfully creamy, go on evenly with good coverage and have good staying potential. The choice of colors is extensive and even the Luminesque, which is too shiny for my personal taste, is a good option if you like a soft pearlized look to your lips. There is a specialty lip product called Triple Action Lip Defense ($5.50). The lipstick tube is striped with a line of blue, pink and white. It does have a Sun Protecting Factor of 19 which is great for the lips, and it is quite emollient, but all the other claims on the package are overstated and contrived. Lip Zone Protector ($7.95) is a two-in-one tube applicator; one end is called Roll-away, the other Fill-in. Roll-away is a white gloss-like cream made up of wax and clay. You place it on the lips, leave it to dry and then rub it off, peeling off a layer of skin as you rub, which supposedly leaves a smooth layer of skin behind. The other end is supposed to fill in the lines around the mouth and prevent lipstick from feathering. It is an interesting concept, but it doesn't work. I found the Roll-Away too irritating for my skin and the fill-in part of the tube didn't keep my lipstick from feathering and it tasted awful. Revlon has a lip-color compact, half of which contains powder and half a lip gloss called Powder-on-Lip-Color ($5.50). The powder goes on first and then the gloss is supposed to go over the powder. This all feels very dry, and the color may still bleed into the lines around the mouth. Lips tend to become dry when you use these powdered lip colors for a period of time. The last in this long line of lip products is Color-Lock ($5.50), an anti-feathering lip product that truly works! You could save yourself a lot of time and trouble and just get the Color-Lock and a few of the Revlon lipsticks and you and your lips would be very happy.

Eye and Brow Pencils: Revlon has several types of eyeliner. One is a pencil called Micro Pure Slimliner ($4.95), which, in spite of its fancy packaging, is just a pencil, but a rather good one at that. Another is a traditional liquid liner called Fabuliner ($4.95) which looks like something I used in the 1960s. The last one is a felt-tip pen applicator called Precision Eyelining Pen ($4.75). I have a hard time recommending any of these. The Fabuliner is a traditional liquid liner that makes a hard line around the eye. The felt-tip eyelining pen goes on somewhat softer than the Fabuliner, but it too makes the eye look "lined." If you want a specific line around your eye, the Fabuliner is as good as any. Because of the packaging, there is no way for you to see the color. The same is true for the pencils, therefore both of them are difficult to recommend. The Waterproof Eyeshaper ($4.25) is basically an acceptable liner, but it tends toward the greasy side and would be better if it weren't waterproof. Because of the greasy texture, you would not want to use this on your eyebrows and if you are concerned at all about eyeliner smearing, this is not a great option. Revlon also has an eyeshadow stick called Powder Pencil ($4.25) that is waterproof as well. It comes in a good selection of colors, but I find it difficult to recommend because it can smear too easily, although it can aid in creating an eye design in a hurry and without mess.

Lip Pencil: Revlon's lip pencils ($4.25) come in a nice assortment of colors and have a wonderful texture. These are waterproof, but given that lipstick is wiped off anyway, there is no problem with it being waterproof. The eyebrow pencils are not the best; one is Waterproof Eyebrow Pencil ($3.50) that goes on fairly dry and hard. The other is an automatic pencil called Color-Up Stick for Brows ($3.75). It is convenient, but extremely greasy and will make the brow look artificial.

Mascara: Revlon makes a specialty eyelash product called Lash Repair ($4.95). It is mostly alcohol and water, which not only won't repair lashes, it will dry them out. There is also a Sheer Tint Mascara that makes little or no difference in the way your lashes look. These sheer-tint products won't last long on the market because they make only a minimal difference in the way your lashes look. If you have lashes that are already black and thick and you want them to have a little more definition, then the clear mascaras are an option to consider. Two of their new mascara's Long Distance Mascara and Quick Thick Mascara ($4.95) are both excellent; no smudging, easy, quick application and they make lashes thick and long.

Brushes: Revlon has several brushes in good shapes and sizes, but the blush brush ($6.50) and eyeshadow brush ($4.25) have oversized handles that are cumbersome and hard to carry in a makeup bag for touchups during the day.

Shiseido

Shiseido is unique in that it is the only Japanese name-brand cosmetics line sold in U.S. department stores. I'm sure part of its sales appeal is the reputation the Japanese have for creating excellent products. I'm not sure that this reputation holds for makeup. I find Shiseido a rather limited makeup line with a limited variety of makeup products. However, some Shiseido products are excellent. I particularly like their lipsticks, which are very creamy. Some of their foundations are also excellent, and the blush colors are quite nice and have a beautiful silky texture. As do many cosmetics lines, Shiseido has an endless array of shiny eyeshadows that make the skin look wrinkly and over-madeup for daytime. The counter displays are attractive, but you need a salesperson to help you with the products, which are all out of the consumer's reach. Most of the salespeople were well trained and knew how to bring up the subject of skin care even when I was only trying on a lipstick.

Foundation: Shiseido makes four types of foundation. Stick Foundation (for dry skin only) goes on fairly greasy, though it can blend to be surprisingly sheer; Fluid Foundation has a great consistency, but a poor selection of colors; Creme Powder Compact Foundation looks like a cream but dries to a silky, light-coverage powder; and Dual Compact Powder ($29) is a pressed powder that can be used wet or dry and comes in an excellent assortment of sheer colors. It is basically a talc and mineral oil powder that is best used as a finishing powder and not a foundation.

Foundation Colors to Try

Stick Foundation ($24)

I2: Great neutral color for fair to medium skin tones.

I4: Great color choice.

B2: Great color choice.

B4: Good color for medium skin tones but can turn orange.

B6: Great color for medium skin tone.

G1: Great bronze color for darker skin tones.

Fluid Foundation ($26)

B2 Natural Light Beige: Good color for fair skin tones.

B6 Natural Deep Beige: Great color choice for medium to dark skin tones.

I4 Natural Fair Ivory: Great color for fair skin tones.

Compact Foundation ($23)

All of these colors are excellent: Natural Light Beige, Natural Fair Beige, Natural Deep Beige, Natural Light Pink, Natural Fair Pink, Natural Deep Pink, Warm Bronze, Natural Light Ivory and Natural Fair Ivory.

Foundation Colors to Avoid

Stick Foundation ($24)

P4: Can turn orange on most skin tones.

P2: Can be too pink-peach for most skin tones.

C1: A green primer color for the skin, something I never recommend using.

Fluid Foundation ($26)

P2 Natural Light Pink: May be too pink for most skin tones.

P4 Natural Fair Pink: Too orange for most skin tones.

P6 Natural Deep Pink: May turn orange on some skin tones.

G1 Warm Bronze: May turn orange on some skin tones.

B4 Natural Fair Beige: May turn orange on some skin tones.

Finishing Powder: Shiseido has a large selection of compact powders ($26) that go on very sheer and contain talc, clay and mineral oil. Nothing special for a fairly steep price tag.

Blush Colors to Try

Singles and Trios ($22/$28)

All the colors are beautiful: Coral Brown (good contour color), Rose Ochre, Brown Beige, Hot Brown (good contour color),

Grape (preferably for darker skin tones), Soft Pink, Brown Red Trio, and Brown Beige Trio.

Eyeshadow Colors to Try

Trio ($25)

Brown Variation: Great combination of brown, amber and gray-brown.

Blue Variations: Beautiful combination of deep navy, charcoal and deep violet.

Immutable Ashes: Great combination of ash-brown, soft violet and gray-brown.

Desert Hues: Shiny, but can be an interesting combination for evening wear.

Eyeshadow Colors to Avoid

Single, Duos and Trios ($18/$21/$25)

All of these colors are extremely shiny: Copper Shell, Shell Pink, Hot Gold, Mauve Pink, White Gold, Celadon, Pure Gold, Crystal Lavender, Shiny Shell, Pink Quartz Nuance, Golden Green Nuance, Azure Nuance, The Anthracites, The Jades, The Indigos, Bronze/Copper, Violet/Rust, The Tortoise Shells, The Purple Quartz, Golden Coral/Rose Coral, Clove/Violet, Brick Tones, Soft Petals, Rose Opal and Pearls & Onyx.

Lipstick: Shiseido's lipstick ($12) has a wonderful creamy texture, with a matte finish that is really beautiful. I like these lipsticks a lot. They also have a small selection of traditional lip glosses that come in lipstick form and are nothing special.

Eye, Lip and Brow Pencils: The lipliners ($11) have an excellent dry texture and come in a lovely array of colors. The eyepencils ($13) have a wonderful texture and come in soft muted colors. The brow pencils go on heavier than most and would need to be blended carefully.

Ultima II

Ultima is one of those rare lines that offers prepackaged samples of almost all their products, including lipsticks and foundations. Thank you, Ultima II. It's a wonderful thing to offer the consumer. Another smart move of Ultima II's is its phasing out of shiny eyeshadows while increasing the selection of matte shadows. Their new matte selections are beautiful and worth a try for almost all skin types and skin tones. Their blushes still have more shine than is really necessary, but some are better than others.

The Ultima II display units are attractive, though you need to ask the salesperson for assistance in order to use any of them. I found the Ultima II sales staff less aggressive than most wherever I went, which made shopping their counters less intimidating. Ultima is definitely a line to consider if subtle or natural is the way you want to look. They have a wide range of lipstick shades that vary from natural to full, bold colors, and the foundations from the New Nakeds product line are excellent. (I've listed the New Nakeds eyeshadows, blushes, and concealers separately.)

The New Nakeds Foundation: Ultima II's foundations are divided into yellow-, pink- and neutral-based tones. Usually I recommend against pink-toned foundations (no one has pink skin), but these pink tones are fairly neutral. I would encourage you to take a look at the New Nakeds foundations. There are two formulas: Oil-Control, and Moisturizing Formula. There is actually little difference between the two (neither contains oil) and both go on well, give medium coverage, feel light, and the color selections are some of the best around. They are rated with a SPF of 6, but that's too low to properly protect you skin from the sun. The cream-to-powder foundation, called Brush-On Foundation, goes on very sheer and comes in a beautiful array of colors. This product applies better with a sponge than it does with the brush that comes in the compact.

Foundation Colors to Try

The New Nakeds Oil-Control ($22.50)

All of these are excellent colors: F1Y, F2P, F3P, F6N, F8Y/N, F9Y, F10N, F11P. F14Y/N and F15Y/N are both excellent colors for darker skin tones.

The New Nakeds Moisturizing Formula ($22.50)
All of these are excellent colors: F1Y, F2P, F3P, F5N, F7Y/N, F8Y/N, F9Y, F10N, F11P, F12Y/N, F13Y/N. F14Y/N and F15Y/N are both excellent color choice for darker skin tones.

Brush-On Foundation ($25)
All of these are beautiful colors: 2Y, 3Y, 1N, 2N, 3N, 1P, 2P and 3P.

Foundation Colors to Avoid

The Nakeds Oil-Control ($22.50)
F4Y: Can be too peach.
F5P: Too peach for most skin tones.
F7Y/N: Too yellow for most skin tones.
F12Y/N: Can turn orange on most skin tones.
F13Y/N: Can be too orange for most skin tones.

The Nakeds Moisturizing Formula ($22.50)
F4Y: Can be too peach for most skin tones.
F6P: Can turn peach on most skin tones.

Finishing Powder: Ultima II has a Loose Powder ($19.50) and a Pressed Powder ($15.50). Both have almost identical talc-based formulas, though the loose powder does have a slight shine added to it. They go on quite sheer and have a nice texture, but they are fairly expensive for what you get. The colors are numbered 1 to 6 and range from almost white to bronze. They also have Rice Powder Compacts ($17) that are very shiny and can be used for evening wear only.

Blush: Unfortunately, most of the Ultima II blushes have some amount of shine — not a lot, but enough to make oily skin look shinier than it already is — they also tend to make dry skin look more dry. Normal skin (without freckles or scarring) can handle shiny blushes better than the other skin types.

Blush Colors to Try

Creamy Powder Blush ($15)
Crystal Rose: Worth a try but slightly shiny.
Porcelain Mauve: Could be a great eyeshadow, not a great blush color for most skin tones.
Pink Sand: A very soft pink.
Hibiscus: A good color.

Grenadine Fizz: Worth a try but slightly shiny.

Bronze Bordeaux: May be too shiny for most skin types.

Sahara Rose: Pretty color, though it does have some shine.

Rose Apricot: Ok color, but probably too shiny for most skin types.

Sheer Currant: Great color.

Sheer Bronze: May be too brown for most skin types, but basically a good color though slightly shiny.

Sheer Peach: Would make a great eyeshadow, though slightly shiny.

Sheer Pink: Slightly shiny.

Blush Colors to Avoid

Creamy Powder Blush ($15)

All of these colors are too shiny: Rose Amethyst, Chestnut Frost, Frosted Honey Umber (evening wear only), Burnished Bordeaux, Ginger Plum Frost and Sheer Orchid.

Eyeshadow Colors to Try

Singles, Duos and Trios ($12.50/$15.50/$18.50)

Chip: Good tan brown.

Disk: Good shade of ash-gray.

Circuit: Deep shade of forest green.

PC: Good shade of navy.

Eyeshadow Colors to Avoid

Singles, Duos and Trios ($12.50/$15.50/$18.50)

Smolder/Flirt/Blush: Flirt may be a bit bright.

Thunder/Cloud/Storm: Too blue for my taste, but if you're for gray/blue tones these are ok.

Black Navy/Chamois/Hematite: Fairly shiny, though nice colors; best for night wear only.

Sable/Fleece/Ochre: For night wear only.

Jungle/Sun: Sun would be used for night only.

Moonlit Orchid/Tropic Moondust: For night wear only; too shiny for daytime.

Indigo Sky/Violet Sky: Violet Sky is too shiny.

Pebble/Sand: Sand is too white, though Pebble is a nice color.

Charcoal/Angora/Black Plum: Angora is too white, and this shade of Charcoal may look blue on some skin tones.

Root/Lichen/Moss: A very difficult combination of colors to use.

Midnight Mauve/Prairie Mauve: Too shiny.

Heather Plum/Spunsilver Mauve: Spunsilver is much too shiny, though Heather Plum is a good color.

Spungold Wine/Wine Mist: Too shiny.

Blue Smoke/Sheer Silver Blue: Sheer Silver is very shiny.

Midnight/Morning: Highly contrasting combination which makes it difficult to use.

Sky/Shell : Too shiny.

Aquamarine/Roseshell: Very bright, contrasting colors make it a difficult combination to use.

Black Emerald/Candlelight: Too shiny.

Almond Cocoa/Spunsilver Beige: Almond is a nice color, but Spunsilver is too shiny.

Mushroom/Peach Sorbet: Too shiny.

Micro: Too white for most skin tones.

Byte : Strange shade of pale green.

The New Nakeds Eyeshadow: This is Ultima II's new matte color line and it is quite impressive. None of the eyeshadows is the least bit shiny. Each goes on smoothly and true. The eyeshadows are particularly well organized from light to dark. I recommend almost all of these.

The New Nakeds Eyeshadows to Try

Singles and Duos ($12/$18.50)

All of these are excellent matte colors: 1 (may be too white for most skin tones); 2, 3, 4, 5, 6 (would make a great eyebrow color), 7, 8, 9 (too white for most skin tones); 10, 11, 12, 13 (very bright green, probably best for redheads or blondes); 14 (too green for my taste, but it could be a decent eyeliner or accent color); 15 (perfect contour color), 16 (great contour color for darker skin tones); 1 & 5 (strong contrast, may be tricky to use); 2 & 6, 3 & 7, 4 & 8 and 8 & 1 (strong contrast, may be tricky to use).

The New Nakeds Cheek Color to Try

All Cheek Colors ($16.50)

All of these are great colors, although they may be too brown for some skin tones: 1, 2, 3, 4, 5 and 6 (a perfect contour color).

The New Nakeds Cheek Color to Avoid
All Cheek Colors ($16.50)
  All of these are too shiny: 7, 8, 9, 10 and 11

Concealer: Ultima II's New Nakeds line has a good selection of concealer and colors. The consistency is smooth without being too dry or too greasy.

Concealer Colors to Try
All Concealer Colors ($11.50)
  C2: May turn pink or orange on some skin tones, but only
      slightly.
  C3: Very good color for dark skin tones only.
  C4: Nice color for dark skin tones only.
  C6: Nice color; even though it is the darkest concealer color, it is
      not a great color for darker skin tones.

Concealer Colors to Avoid
All Concealer Colors ($11.50)
  C1: May turn pink on most skin tones.
  C5: Too orange for almost all skin tones.

Lipstick: Ultima II has several types of lipstick with a wide range of color choices. There are Mattes ($11), Lip Chrome ($13) and Super Luscious ($11). Most of these have excellent textures and go on in a variety of consistencies from creamy to extremely dry.

Lip, Eye and Brow Pencils: The eye and brow pencils ($12.50) are somewhat greasy, so they smudge well, but can also smear. One end of the pencil has a sponge tip to help soften lines after application. Do not use these on the eyebrow or they will appear shiny because of the greasier formula. Ultima II also has an Eyebrow Gel ($12.50) that is quite good and doesn't go on too heavy, but it only comes in a clear gel and an ash-brown color, a rather limited selection. The Lip Pencils ($9) come in a nice variety of colors, have a smooth texture, but are not outstanding.

Victoria Jackson

Victoria Jackson Cosmetics is a complete line of makeup and skin care products sold on television via very slick, half-hour info-commercials. I am strongly opposed to buying makeup that you can neither try on or see and instead have to base your decision on television sales techniques. The reason I chose to include this line was based in large part on curiosity: I wanted to see for myself if the claims in the ads were valid. Plus it was hard to ignore the apparent popularity of this commercial. I called their 1-800 number and was connected to a clearing house of operators that are used for many "call-in-now" type products. I was asked a couple of questions—my skin tone (light, medium, tan or dark) and what colors did I prefer (red, peach or pink) — I answered medium and red. After being given two payment options, I was told my products would be delivered in four to six weeks. Two weeks later my package arrived.

Almost everything you would need to do a complete makeup application and cleansing routine (skin care products are reviewed in Chapter 7) was sent in the introductory kit. The makeup items included a brush set (no sponge-tips), four eyeshadows, two shades of foundation in one compact, a retractable lip pencil, three retractable eye or brow pencils, 4 shades of lip color that come in a compact, two blushers, pressed translucent powder, mascara and lash conditioner, a packet of instruction cards, an instructional video tape and reorder forms. Quite a kit. Total price, $125.85. Each item in the kit was marked at a higher price than what I actually paid. For example, the foundation was marked at $24.95, although I received the "special" price of $12.95 that was listed on the order form. All the Victoria Jackson products have two price categories. If you order $20 or more worth of products, you can get the cheaper price everytime. This is a cosmetic line that likes making deals. But what about the products?

The makeup items I received, for the most part, were fine, although nothing special and a few of the products didn't work well at all. This isn't a very complicated line. The limitations make ordering easier, but the drawback is that fewer options can't really accommodate a lot of different skin tones or color preferences (although you are encouraged to mix the colors together to achieve a wider range of colors). There are three other groupings of colors called Morning, Noon and Night that weren't available as this book went to press.)

The makeup demonstration video tape that came with the introductory kit was very interesting. I didn't always agree with Victoria's application techniques. For example, she recommends applying eyeliner and brow color before the eyeshadows which would undo or mess up the eyebrow you created and the liner you applied. Those are minor points; basically this is a good, understandable makeup video. The problem I had with the tape is that 50 percent of it made me feel as if I was sitting through another television ad, listening to Victoria and a guest celebrity talk about how great the products are. I already bought the products, now I wanted to learn more about how to use them. I suppose that sometimes it's hard to stop selling when you have to pay for expensive television time.

Foundation: Victoria Jackson has one type of foundation ($24.95/ $12.95) that comes in a single compact with two shades for each of four categories of skin tones: light, medium, tan and dark. The colors are good, though the medium shades are a tad on the ashy-green side and the light is a bit pink. In order to create the right color for you, you are supposed to mix the two colors together, which is fine if you know how to mix the right proportions. If you don't, you're likely to have trouble. I found the foundation to be quite thick and I would not call the application sheer as the commercial claims. It is a petrolatum based foundation and therefore somewhat greasy. Oily or combination skins would not be happy with this one.

Concealer: There is no individually packed concealer in the Victoria Jackson line. The suggestion is to use the lightest shade of foundation in the dual foundation compact for the undereye area. This would be a great idea if the foundation weren't so greasy. It easily fills into the lines under the eye and any liner you then place around the eye will probably smear.

Finishing Powder: The pressed compact powders ($16.95/$8.95) come in four shades: light, medium, tan and dark, and are talc-based. The colors are all fine and the textures sheer and light.

Blush: Each color family kit (peach, red and pink) comes with a blush compact ($19.95/$9.95) that contains two colors. One of the colors is always a light pale shade of peachy-pink and the other a more vivid color. The textures and colors are very good. The red kit's blush color is a nice shade of coral (which is not red by the way); the pink kit's blush color is a soft shade of pink; and the peach kit's is a brown-peach shade which is probably too brown for most skin tones.

Eyeshadow: The eyeshadow sets ($19.95/$9.95) come in a single compact of four different colors. The color combinations are excellent; unfortunately almost all are slightly shiny.

Lipstick: Victoria Jackson includes a lipstick compact ($17.94/$8.95) in each color kit that contains three shades of lip creams and a lip color powder. The colors are fine, but the lip creams are very greasy and if you have any problem with bleeding lipstick, these are not for you. The lip powder is a problem because it tends to cake on the lips and dry them out when used alone or over an extended period of time. There are lipstick colors listed on the order sheet that come in tubes, but there are no color swatches provided to assist in making a decision.

Lip, Eye and Brow Pencils: All of the pencils ($7.95/$4) in the introductory kit are retractable and have a great texture. There are three eye or brow pencils in each kit; black, chocolate brown and taupe; and a lip pencil that matches the color categories of peach, pink and red. They are all great, and at the $4 price, an excellent buy.

Mascara: Every introductory kit comes packaged with a dual black mascara ($12.95/$6.50): one end is a clear conditioner; the other black mascara. The mascara is good but the conditioner is mostly a plastic-like substance and glycerin; it won't do much for the lashes and I didn't notice a difference whether I used it or not. Victoria Jackson's traditional black mascara ($13.95/$7.94) is great just by itself.

Brushes: Victoria Jackson includes a set of brushes in the introductory kit that are adequate but not great: a retractable brush set ($40/$24.95) that includes a retractable blush brush and retractable lip brush is overpriced at either cost; and a professional brush set ($18.95/$9.50) that includes a lip brush, eyebrow brush/comb, two-sided eyeshadow brush and a blush brush. The brushes have sparse hair and are not firm enough to hold the color well. These brushes are useful, but there are better ones on the market.

Comment from woman who creates labels for cosmetics:

"It takes a lot of work to make something sound true when it isn't and not get in trouble with the FDA!"

CHAPTER SEVEN

Evaluation of the Major Cosmetics Companies' Skin Care Products

THE PROCESS

I have one confession to make before I begin my analysis of skin care products: This section of the book has been the most difficult to write because I truly find almost all the skin care products at the cosmetics counters to be absurdly overpriced and many of their claims, outrageous. Don't get me wrong — there are decent products at the cosmetics counters. There are cleansers that clean the face without leaving the skin greasy or dry, toners that exfoliate the skin without irritating it and moisturizers that alleviate dry skin. It's just that I find the hoopla, hyperbole and expense impossible to consider without groaning in exasperation and anger. Just to set the record straight: Anything you can buy at the department store cosmetics counters, you can buy for much less at the drugstore, and the product will be just as effective. It's not so hard to believe once you realize that many of the drugstore products contain many of the same ingredients as similar items carried in department stores. Furthermore, many fancy department store lines are frequently owned by the same parent company who makes the drugstore products: Revlon owns Borghese, Alexandra de Markoff, Max Factor and Ultima II; Cosmair owns L'Oreal and Lancome; and Chesebrough Ponds owns Erno Lazlo and Aziza. There are many enticing advertisements that will persuade you to spend $30, $50 or more on a moisturizer, but I just want it to be perfectly clear what a waste of money I think that is.

The extensive inventory being recommended at the cosmetics counters to close pores, smooth skin, eliminate wrinkles via exfoliation, balance the pH of the skin and generally rejuvenate the face is nothing less than astonishing. In addition is an array of products the face from the sun and counteract its negative effects. Regardless of the product, each salesperson I talked to was deeply earnest about how it would vastly improve my skin if I used it. The formulations were all described as superior — nothing less than miraculous. Every product was promoted as having been tested and certified by the proper scientific authorities and, besides, the salesperson was always using it herself and couldn't do without it. Although very little of what I heard ever made any sense, it always sounded so convincing. I can only imagine how hard it must be for a consumer not to believe what is proposed when it comes to the products they need to take care of their skin.

How someone decides what to buy has always been a wonder to me. We scrutinize the contents of a $1.75 box of cereal we're thinking of buying for tomorrow morning's breakfast, yet, ironically, most consumers have no idea what is actually in their cosmetics. They nevertheless spend quite a bit of money on a series of items that they know very little about. I suspect it is easy to lose perspective when the subject is as personal and frustrating as skin care. Perhaps one of the only ways to eliminate the emotional charge from this issue, and to protect our budget at the same time, is to evaluate skin care products from a more objective frame of reference. Fortunately, the cosmetics companies have provided us with the very tool we need to implement such a criteria — the ingredient label.

Every skin care item (and makeup item for that matter) lists the contents on the box or container. This ingredient list can be your best friend because it can't mislead you. The information there, by law, has to be accurate. Every skin care product I reviewed was evaluated on the basis of what it contained. You will have to test for yourself how it feels on your skin. My mission was simply to compare the promises made about a particular product to the ingredients listed on the label. Whatever the claim, the ingredients are the basis for whether or not a claim can be verified.

The question I asked myself as I examined each item was simple: Is this product substantially different from other similar products out on the market? If all eye makeup removers have essentially the same ingredients, does it make sense to buy one that costs $17 or $5? Or if a $50 wrinkle cream is essentially the same as a $10 wrinkle cream, does it make sense to spend the $50? To establish that point, I've listed each products specific, key ingredients so that you can begin to familiarize yourself with the repetitive nature of cosmetic formulations.

As you go through the list of products you will notice that I did not review every product each line carries. I reviewed the products that I felt were most representative of that particular line. I chose not to review many sunscreen or sun-related products, because there is no real difference in the effectiveness of sunscreens which have the same SPF number. If your sunscreen has an SPF factor of 15 or greater, that's what counts the most. Avoid sunscreens that contain irritating ingredients such as alcohol or witch hazel. Except for those, all sunscreens with the same SPF factor essentially do the same job — even the cheap ones.

When it came to facial cleansers, I was interested primarily in how genuinely water-soluble they were. I expected facial cleansers to rinse off easily without the aid of a washcloth. Once a water-soluble cleanser is rinsed off, it should also not leave a greasy, filmy feeling to the skin. Although I never recommend cold cream-type cleansers, I included some of them for your information. If a cleanser was designed for oily skin, then I wanted to know how gentle or irritating it was on the skin. I expected all facial cleansers to be able to remove eye makeup as well as face makeup without being greasy or drying. I do not feel it is be necessary to use a second product, such as an eye makeup remover, to do what the facial cleanser should be doing all by itself. Because I feel that using an eye makeup removers is an extraneous step, I included those products for those of you who feel that this method is indispensable. I also did not include bar soaps in my review because of their tendency to dry out the skin. Too many problems occur when cleansers of any kind either dry out the skin or make it too greasy. I explain my skin care concepts in Chapter Four, and, in more detail, in *Blue Eyeshadow Should Still Be Illegal.*

I never recommend astringents, toners and fresheners that contain irritating ingredients of any kind such as alcohol, acetone, witch hazel or citrus juices such as grapefruit or orange. These products were evaluated on that basis alone. Claims of closing pores or refining the skin are not realistic, so I was looking primarily for astringents, toners and fresheners that left a smooth, soft feeling to the face, without any irritation whatsoever.

As you already know by now, there is no such thing as a "legitimate" wrinkle cream — a potion that can permanently eliminate wrinkles. There are moisturizers that can temporarily improve dry skin and some are indeed fabulous. Actually, almost all the moisturizers and wrinkle creams I reviewed take care of dry skin beautifully. Wrinkle creams and moisturizers from my view point are all one-in-the-same and I expected the same thing from all of them: They must contain ingredients that can smooth dry skin. I indicated which products contained some of the latest moisturizing ingredients that are thought to be effective such as: Hyaluronic acid, sodium pca, proteins and collagen (see Chapter Two for more specifics). In addition, I listed the ingredients that I thought were more hype than proven moisturizing agents. Many cosmetics lines include every new ingredient on the market just so they can claim to contain anything and everything that may have some impact on dry skin. Often the percentage of these ingredients in a product is so small that it is practically insignificant.

When you check the ingredient list of a product, you should realize that the first five to ten ingredients — the one most abundant in the formulas — are those that effect your skin the greatest. Ingredient labels are organized in descending order. The most used ingredient is listed first, the next most used is listed second and so on. For the most part, the ingredients I listed for each product follows the sequential order in which they appear on the product's ingredient label. In the listing below, when I describe each skin care item, I frequently cite the first five ingredients either by name or description, to assist you in understanding how I evaluated the product. (For further information regarding ingredient descriptions, please refer to Ruth Winter's *A Consumer's Dictionary of Cosmetic Ingredients,* Third Edition.)

It is also important to remember that a moisturizer containing an SPF of less than 15 is not considered adequate to truly protect the skin from the sun. Most moisturizers that indicate they contain a sunscreen but do not indicate an SPF rating, usually only contain only an SPF of 4 or 6.

Facial masks are a group of products that contain mostly clay-like ingredients. They absorb oil and, to some degree, help exfoliate the skin. The problem with many of these products is that they can be too irritating for most skin types. Although your face may initially feel smooth when the mask is first rinsed off, after a short period of time, the drying effect it has on the skin creates problems. You want to shun facial masks that contain drying or irritating ingredients in addition to the clay component: Masks that contain camphor, alcohol, menthol, eucalyptus and benzyl peroxide should all be avoided. Clay masks that contain emollients and moisturizing ingredients may be satisfactory for dry skin, but can cause oily skin to breakout.

Note: *Although the cost of cosmetics often fluctuates, I've included prices solely for the sake of comparison. When two prices are listed for the same product, the first one is for the smaller size, the second for the larger.*

And so, the results of my evaluations are listed below in alphabetical order by company:

Adrien Arpel

Freeze-Dried Embryonic Collagen Protein Cleanser *($19.50):* I'm of the opinion that freeze-dried embryonic collagen, which is tissue from an animal fetus, is useless. This cleanser is otherwise satisfactory, although a bit on the greasy side.

Sea Kelp Cleanser *($18.50):* This cleanser is a scrub that is fairly greasy and will not rinse off without the aid of a washcloth. In addition to the particles of sea kelp and salt, it contains mineral oil and petrolatum.

Coconut Cleanser *($16.50):* This cleanser contains mostly water, safflower oil and propylene glycol. It will not rinse off without the aid of a washcloth.

Honey Almond Scrub *($18.50/$28):* This scrub contains glycerin, almonds and thickeners. It will help slough skin, although baking soda, mixed with a little water, will do the same thing.

Lemon & Lime Freshener *($16.50):* This alcohol-free freshener contains water, propylene glycol, aloe, pectin, vitamin C, and rose hips. It can be soothing and slightly cooling to normal to oily skin types without being irritating.

Herbal Astringent *($16.50):* There is no alcohol in this astringent, although it contains mostly propylene glycol, polysorbate and preservatives. Its claim to close pores for any real length of time is not possible.

Bio Cellular Night Cream *($34.50/$49.50):* This is a very emollient, rich moisturizer containing mineral oil and lanolin. It also contains hydrogenated tallow which can be a skin sensitizer.

Swiss Formula Day Cream #12 *($28/$46):* This is a very emollient, although somewhat lightweight moisturizer. It contains water, propylene glycol, mineral oil, collagen and lanolin. It claims to be not non-greasy, but that doesn't jive with the inclusion of mineral oil and lanolin, both fairly greasy ingredients.

Vital Velvet Moisturizer *($20):* This moisturizer contains mostly water, propylene glycol, lanolin and mineral oil. This is a fairly emollient moisturizer and works well for extremely dry skin only.

Moisturizing Blotting Lotion *($19.50):* This moisturizer does not contain oil; rather, it contains clay that is supposed to absorb oil and emollients to improve of dry skin. Unfortunately, even though there is no oil in this product, the emollients can cause breakouts. Unless you're using other products that dry out your skin, you don't need a moisturizer if you have oily skin.

Morning After Moisturizer, SPF 20 *($30):* This intriguingly named product is a good, basic, lightweight moisturizer, with a high SPF number, which makes it a good sunscreen.

Almay

Moisture Balance Cleansing Lotion for Normal Skin *($7):* This is a very emollient cleanser that does not rinse off without the aid of a washcloth. If you have normal skin, you will find this cleanser somewhat greasy.

Deep Cleansing Cold Cream *($3.55):* This cleanser is a traditional cold cream that needs to be wiped off and will leave the skin feeling greasy.

Oil Control Cleansing Lotion *($7):* This cleanser lathers nicely but can be very drying and irritating to the skin. It may also burn the eyes.

Sensitive Skin Cleanser *($6.50):* Like many cleansers, this one contains a gentle detergent usually found in shampoos. I found it to be too drying on my skin, although it did rinse off easily.

Moisture Renew Balance Toner for Dry Skin *($7):* This product contains mostly water and alcohol and can irritate the skin.

Moisture Balance Toner for Normal Skin *($7):* This product contains ingredients almost identical to the toner above and it too can irritate the skin.

Oil Control Toner for Oily Skin *($7):* This toner contains ingredients almost identical as the two previously mentioned toners and is similarly irritating to the skin.

Oil Relief Gel *($9.50):* This moisturizer is recommended for oily skin and contains mostly water, alcohol, butylene glycol and allantoin. What moisture you gain from the other ingredients is negated by the drying effect of the alcohol.

Stress Cream *($7.50):* This cream contains good moisturizing ingredients and many of the latest components designed to keep water in the skin.

It is a fine moisturizer that contains mostly water, propylene glycol, mineral oil, butylene glycol, a glycerin-like ingredient and petrolatum. The product can't counteract stress as the name implies, but it will improve dry skin.

Stress Eye Gel *($7.50):* This lightweight gel contains an interesting assortment of ingredients that include water, a gel-like ingredient, butylene glycol, an amino acid, allantoin, aloe vera gel, hyaluronic acid and sodium pca. All these should feel soothing around the eye and keep moisture in the skin without leaving it feeling greasy. Unfortunately, this product also contains witch hazel which can be too irritating for the delicate skin around the eye.

Moisture Renew Cream for Dry Skin *($6.50):* This lightweight moisturizer contains water, mineral oil, propylene glycol, thickeners and sodium pca. It is a good moisturizer although it would be better for normal to dry skin. It doesn't contain enough emollients to really soothe extremely dry skin.

Moisture Balance Eye Cream for Normal Skin *($5):* This very rich cream works better for extremely dry skin than it would for normal skin. It contains petrolatum, lanolin oil, mineral oil, propylene glycol, water and paraffin.

Moisture Renew Lotion for Dry Skin *($8):* This lightweight moisturizer is similar to the cream, but in lotion form.

The Body Shop

As I explained in Chapter Six, there are many things about The Body Shop that I admire. For example, their products come in recyclable containers and the shop's bags read: "The question is not, can they reason? Nor, can they talk? But, can they suffer?" This company stands by its principles every step of the way. I wish I had the same positive feelings about their skin care products, but I don't. Their water-soluble cleansers don't rinse off without the aid of a washcloth, the toners contain irritating ingredients such as alcohol and some of their moisturizers contain ingredients that can cause blackheads. Additionally, several of their products also contain the preservative 2-bromo-2-nitropane-1, 3 diol and a water softener called triethanolamine. When these two ingredients are present in the same cosmetic they can be very irritating, and even dangerous, on your skin. There is also an increased chance of having an allergic reaction to products that contain herbs and flowers. If you have hayfever, you are a prime candidate for having skin that will react to these kind of products. One quality I do like about The Body Shop's skin care line is that the company makes few — if any — exaggerated claims as to what its products can and can't do for the skin. Now that's a refreshing change from what you will find in almost every other cosmetics line. You can also buy small, very inexpensive samples of their skin care products.

Note: *There are four different sizes of most every skin care product at The Body Shop. The prices listed below are for the 8.4-ounce size only.*

Cucumber Cleansing Milk *($8.15):* This cleanser contains mostly water, glycerin, mineral oil, thickeners, cucumber extract and lanolin. It must be wiped off with either a washcloth or tissue. It definitely leaves a greasy residue on the skin. This product also contains 2-bromo-2-nitropane-1, 3 diol and triethanolamine which can be dangerous for the skin.

Passion Fruit Cleansing Gel *($8.15):* The sudsing agent in this cleanser can be irritating to the skin and burn the eyes.

Orchid Oil Cleansing Milk *($8.15):* The main ingredients in this cleanser are water, rosewater, sweet almond oil and oil of orchid. This cleanser must be wiped off with a washcloth or tissue and leaves a greasy residue on the skin.

Orange Flower Water *($8.55):* This toner contains orange flower water and preservatives. It can be soothing, but the amount of preservatives in this product can also be irritating to the skin.

Elderflower Water *($8.55):* This toner contains water, alcohol, castor oil and elderflower extract. The alcohol makes it too irritating for most skin types.

Honey Water *($8.55):* This toner contains rosewater and preservatives. It can be soothing, but the amount of preservatives in this product can also be irritating to the skin.

Aloe Vera Moisture Cream *($7.75):* This rich cream contains water, almond oil, glycerin, cocoa butter, thickeners and aloe vera extract. It should take good care of very dry skin.

Carrot Moisture Cream *($9.40):* This moisturizer is also only for skin types that do not breakout. The second ingredient in this cream is isopropyl myristate which can cause blackheading. Otherwise, this is a lightweight cream that contains water, almond oil, glycerin, thickeners and carrot oil.

Jojoba Moisture Cream *($12.10):* This moisturizer is only for skin types that do not breakout. The second ingredient in this cream is isopropyl myristate which can cause blackheading. Other than that, this is a rich cream that contains water, jojoba oil, wheatgerm oil, thickener and glycerin.

Sage Comfrey Open Pore Cream *($7.75):* This product is mostly water, alcohol, witch hazel and comfrey and sage extract. The alcohol and witch hazel make it too irritating for most skin types.

Glycerin & Rosewater Lotion *($11):* This moisturizer is only for skin types that do not breakout. The second ingredient in this cream is isopropyl myristate which can cause blackheading. Other than that, this lightweight, emollient moisturizer contains water, mineral oil, polawax, glycerin and wheatgerm oil.

White Musk Lotion *($11):* This lightweight, emollient moisturizer contains water, sweet almond oil, coconut oil, thickener, cocoa butter and glycerin. It should work well for dry skin.

Aloe Lotion *($11):* This rich, extremely emollient moisturizer contains aloe vera gel, water, wheatgerm oil, apricot kernel oil, polawax and sodium pca.

Borghese

Crema Saponetta *(Clarifying Cleansing Creme, $26):* This product is mostly water, alcohol, talc, propylene glycol and flower oils. The minerals included are primarily salt, potassium, magnesium, calcium, chloride, and bromide. Because of the alcohol and the minerals, this is probably too irritating for most skin types, although salt is a good "deep cleanser." However, you can add salt or baking soda to almost any water-soluble cleanser and get the same result. There is absolutely no nutritional benefit or any other proven benefit derived from these mineral salts when applied on the skin.

Tonico Minerale *(Stimulating Tonic, $22.50):* This toner contains mostly water, talc, propylene glycol, witch hazel, mineral salts and flower oils. It should feel soothing to most skin types, although dry or normal skin types may find it too drying because of the talc, witch hazel and mineral salts.

Cura di Vita *(Restorative Fluid for Face, $37.50):* This product contains an SPF of 4 to 6 which is not high enough to protect the face effectively from the sun. It primarily contains water, butylene and propylene glycol, thickeners, mineral salts and many of the latest ingredients for keeping moisture in the skin, such as sodium pca and hyaluronic acid. It is a good moisturizer for normal to slightly dry skin.

Cura di Vita Day Fluid *($37.50):* This cream is almost identical to the one above, only it has a thicker consistency.

Restorative Eye Cream *($27.50):* This cream contains water, propylene glycol, a thickener, an oil derived from coconut oil, more thickeners and a form of squalene (shark oil). It also contains a component of nucleic acid and mineral salts. Borghese claims these ingredients do a lot for the skin in terms of "reversing the signs of aging," but I disagree. In spite of false claims it is still a good lightweight moisturizer.

Moisture Intensifier *($65):* This moisturizer primarily contains water, a form of mineral oil, butylene glycol, mineral oil, propylene glycol, mineral salts and flower oils. This is a lot of money for a very basic lightweight moisturizer. It doesn't even contain any of the latest fad moisturizing ingredients.

Concentrato di Vita *($60):* Many cosmetics lines include "special treatments" that come in small vials and are supposed to produce amazing results in a short period of time. Concentrato di Vita is one element in one such system. This attractively packaged, very expensive product contains mostly water mineral oil, isopropyl myristate (which can cause blackheads), propylene glycol and minerals like salt, potassium, calcium and a few others. It does contain some good moisturizing ingredients, but they are so far down in the ingredient list that I can't recommend the product as a good moisturizer.

Fango *($50):* The brochure for this jar of clay described it as "Fango Therapy of Montecantini." Montecantini is supposedly some kind of special volcanic clay. The product actually contains water, bentonite (a white clay found in the United States) and Montecantini clay. It also contains some salt, potassium, magnesium, calcium and some lavender and geranium oil. It does feel good when you take it off, but that's about it, and dry skin types may find the drying effects of the clay too irritating. As a side note, the special clay from Italy isn't even the main type of mud used, although clay from the good old U.S.A. is the second ingredient. Regardless of whose clay it is, this is a lot of money for mud. Period.

Chanel

Demaquillant Fluide *(Cleansing Milk, $27.50):* This cleanser contains mostly water, mineral oil and butylene glycol. It is indeed lightweight, but it won't rinse off easily without help of a washcloth. It also contains isopropyl myristate which can cause blackheads.

Demaquillant Aquapurifiant *(Purifying Clay Cleanser, $23.50):* This cleanser contains water, clay, propylene glycol, mineral oil and a foaming agent. Clay is not the best ingredient for a cleanser because it is hard to rinse off and you wouldn't want to use it over the eye area. And why include mineral oil in a product that is meant to absorb excess oil.

Demaquillant Fraicheur *(Gentle Cleansing Bar, $22.50):* Like most cleansing bars this product contains soap and wax. It also contains dextrin and corn starch, both of which are considered to be potential skin irritants.

Lotion Vivifiante *(Refining Toner, $27.50):* This liquid contains fairly standard ingredients for an alcohol-based toner: water, alcohol, witch hazel and rose water. It is probably too irritating for most skin types.

Lotion Douce *(Firming Freshener — $27.50):* This freshener doesn't contain alcohol, which is good. The main ingredients are water, sorbitol (like glycerin), propylene glycol and lanolin oil. It should feel nice on dry skin, if you are not allergic to lanolin.

Hydra Systeme Maximum Moisturizing Lotion *($32.50/$42.50):* This moisturizer contains an SPF of 8 (which isn't enough to protect you from the sun), water, butylene glycol and a good skin soothing agent. There are also two moisturizing ingredients that are supposed to be unique to Chanel. I found no information to suggest these do anything other than retain moisture in the skin, which is good, but not unique.

Creme-Gel Pour Le Contour Des Yeux *(Firming Eye Cream, $40):* This eye cream contains water, rose water, oil and a lanolin derivative. It is a very rich moisturizer, but there is nothing in this cream that can "firm" the skin.

Creme Extreme Protection *($55):* A good, basic sunscreen with an SPF of 15.

Creme No. 1 *(Skin Recovery Cream, $85/$130):* I've been told that "recovery" is attributed to the second ingredient in this cream which is amniotic fluid. I would disagree with any claims about amniotic fluid doing anything special for the skin. The other ingredients are fairly standard: water, propylene glycol, protein and oil. It is a good moisturizer, but not because of the amniotic fluid. The price is what you would really need to recover from.

Prevention Serum *($50):* This product contains a good sunscreen with an SPF of 15, water, glycerin, propylene glycol and ingredients to make it look like a cream. This is a lot of money for a fairly basic sunscreen. Its claim to be recommended by the Skin Cancer Foundation is not unique — all sunscreens with a high SPF rating are recommended by most medical associations.

Lift Serum *($50):* The company's claims: "Independent tests confirm up to 45 percent reduction in the appearance of visible lines and wrinkles after one months regular use." They follow with a surprisingly honest assertion: "Each skin is different. You may achieve lesser or even greater results." Greater results can probably happen if your skin is totally parched and you've never used a moisturizer before in your life; but then the results would be the same, no matter what moisturizer you used.

Christian Dior

Cleansing Emulsion *($32.50):* Basically water, propylene glycol, thickeners and oil. It will clean the face, but it won't rinse well.

Hydra-Dior Lait Demaquillant *(Skin Cleanser, $32.50):* This cleanser contains lanolin which makes it very difficult to rinse off without use of a washcloth.

Eye Makeup Remover Gel *($17):* This gel contains solvents which can indeed cut through makeup: water, polysorbate 80 and peg 20 methyl glucose sesquisterate.

Eye Makeup Remover *($17):* This liquid contains mostly water, flower water and glycerin. It will take off eye makeup.

Hydra-Dior Lotion Purifiante *($32.50):* This astringent is mostly water and alcohol, which is too irritating for almost all skin types.

Skin Freshener *(for dry skin, $32.50):* This tonic contains water, rose water, witch hazel, propylene glycol and more flower-based waters. The claim is that the particular "flower waters" do special things for the skin. For

$32.50, elderberry and cornflower better do just that. However, for dry skin, I would consider the witch hazel too irritating.

Hydra-Dior Creme Contour Des Yeux *(Eye Creme, $60):* The claim is that this product can "delay the formation of wrinkles." The Federal Drug Administration might take issue with this kind of statement; I know I do. Unless it contains a sunscreen with an SPF of 15 or greater there is no way this claim can be scientifically substantiated.

Moisturizing Day Cream *($58):* This is a lightweight moisturizer that contains mostly water, ppg-2 myristyl ether (makes creams feel silky) mineral oil and glycerin. It also contains a sunscreen, but one not strong enough to protect the skin from the sun.

Revitalizing Cream *($74):* This moisturizer contains mostly water, squalene (shark liver), thickeners, mineral oil and some of the latest moisturizing ingredients further down in the ingredient list. This is a good moisturizer, but the $74 price tag is hard to swallow.

Complexe Liposomes *(for eyes, $32.50):* This moisturizer contains mostly water, glycerin and animal thymus extract. I like liposomes as a skin care ingredient, although there are much less expensive moisturizers on the market that contain the same thing. Animal thymus extract has no proven abilities to do anything special for the skin, but it may simply sound good on the label.

Throat Cream *($54):* This moisturizer doesn't contain anything unique that would make it better for the neck than for your face or elbows. It does contain a sunscreen, but it isn't strong enough to protect your neck from the sun.

Clinique

Crystal Clear Cleansing Oil *($11):* This wipe-off cleanser contains mostly mineral oil. The salesperson said it wouldn't leave an oily residue on my face, although it felt oily to me.

Extremely Gentle Cleansing Cream *($9.50/$17.50):* This cleanser is a traditional cold cream product (requires wiping off) that contains mostly mineral oil, water and beeswax.

Quick Dissolve Makeup Solvent *($14.50):* This makeup remover contains mostly water, mineral oil and propylene glycol. The recommendation is that you are supposed to use this water-soluble cleanser to take off your makeup before you use soap. Two products to clean the face always seems like one too many to me. If soap cleans your face this is an unnecessary step or if the Makeup Solvent cleans your face then you shouldn't need the soap. If you can't use the soap over your eyes, then a water-soluble cleanser that works over the entire face would be the fastest and easiest way to clean your face. Besides, the Makeup Solvent did not feel water-soluble to me.

Eye Makeup Solvent Liquid *($10):* This product contains mostly water, a makeup solvent and butylene glycol. It will take off eye makeup and leaves no greasy residue.

Clean-Up Stick *($9.50):* This is an interesting way to clean-up leftover makeup, or makeup mistakes, but a cotton swab and a moisturizer or cleanser will do the same thing — for a lot less money.

7 Day Scrub Cream *(large size, $14.50):* This scrub product contains mostly mineral oil, water, beeswax, sodium borate (antiseptic) and ozokerite (wax-like thickener). This is a very thick, heavy product that can cause the same problems it's trying to eliminate, because beeswax and ozokerite can cause skin to breakout.

Clarifying Lotion 1, 2, 3 and 4 *(large sizes, $14.50):* All of these lotions contain varying degrees of alcohol, which is very irritating to the skin. Clarifying Lotion 3 also contains salicylic acid and acetone which can create additional irritation. Clarifying Lotion 4 is even stronger than the first three. All of these are too irritating to recommend.

Alcohol-Free Clarifier *($13.50):* I'm fairly certain that Clinique made this Clarifier to compensate for their alcohol-laden Clarifying Lotions 1, 2, 3 and 4. It is very gentle and will leave the skin feeling smooth.

Dramatically Different Moisturizing Lotion *(4 ounces, $18.50):* This moisturizer contains mostly water, mineral oil, sesame oil and propylene glycol. For normal to dry skin this is a good, basic lightweight moisturizer, although it isn't all that "dramatically different" from other moisturizers on the market.

Advanced Care Moisturizer *($32.50):* This moisturizer contains mostly water, thickeners, petrolatum and butylene glycol. The literature calls it a "youth-keeper." It won't keep youth in the skin, but it is a reliable moisturizer for very dry skin.

Sub-Skin Cream *(large size, $38.50)*: The first ingredients are water, collagen extract, thickeners, squalene (shark oil) and butylene glycol. A very good moisturizer, but it won't tighten or firm the skin; it will just keep dry skin at bay.

Daily Eye Benefits *($25)*: This cream contains water, cucumber extract, ivy extract, glycerin and thickeners. The cucumber and ivy are supposed to reduce puffiness around the eye. It didn't help the puffiness around my eyes. I would suppose a slice of cucumber should do the same thing, but then it too doesn't.

Cover Girl

Noxzema *($5)*: The major product Cover Girl makes that I have for years taken issue with is Noxzema. This product contains highly irritating ingredients. At one time, it was advertised as good for sensitive skin. None of the ingredients, which include camphor, phenol, menthol and eucalyptus, would ever be appropriate for sensitive skin, or anyone's skin for that matter.

Elizabeth Arden

Visible Difference Deep Cleansing Lotion *($17.50)*: This is a good, water-soluble cleanser that lathers. It can be drying to the skin and may burn your eyes.

Visible Difference Refining Toner *($15)*: Mostly water, witch hazel, alcohol and glycerin. Too irritating for most skin types.

Revitalizing Tonic *(Millennium Line, $21)*: Contains mostly water and alcohol. Too irritating for most skin tones.

Visible Difference Refining Moisturizer *(large size, $15)*: Contains water, emulsifying wax, glycerin, isopropyl myristate, squalene (shark oil) and beeswax. This is a fairly heavy, thick moisturizer. Can cause blackheads.

Ceramide Time Complex Capsules *($155 for 60 capsules)*: Several salespeople told me, "If women could eat this they would." These plastic foam capsules are more hype then anything else. The ingredients inside that are credited with near miracles are neural lipids extract, epidermal lipid extract and retinyl palmitate. The extracts sound good, but won't do anything beyond that. Retinyl palmitate is a good ingredient, but it has nothing to do with Retin-A.

Day Renewal Emulsion *($45):* The first ingredients in this moisturizer are water, squalene (shark oil), propylene glycol, thickener and lanolin oil. This is a very rich, emollient moisturizer that should be used only for dry skin. If you have a tendency to breakout, stay away from this one.

Eye Renewal Cream *($30):* This is a very rich, thick moisturizer that contains water, mineral oil and lanolin. It will take care of dry skin, but if you are allergic to lanolin, it will cause you problems.

Estee Lauder

Instant Action Rinse-Off Cleanser *($16.50):* This cleanser does not rinse off easily without the use of a washcloth. The cleansing agent is mild, so this product can be good for dry skin.

Facewash Self-Foaming System *($16.50):* The second ingredient in this cleanser is tea-lauryl sulfate, which is a fairly strong shampoo-type cleansing agent. It can burn your eyes and make your skin feel dry.

Rich Results *(Hydrating Cleanser, $20):* This cleanser contains a gentle cleansing agent, but it also contains mineral oil and other oils that make it hard to rinse off without the aid of a washcloth.

Re-Nutriv Extremely Delicate Cleanser *($30):* This cleanser is more like a traditional cold cream than anything else. The very greasy formula contains mineral oil, water, beeswax, petrolatum and squalene (shark oil).

Gentle Protection Tonic *(alcohol-free, $22.50):* This is a fairly mild skin toner with very soothing ingredients, including allantoin and ammonium glycyrrhizinate (which doesn't sound soothing, but it is). It does contain horse chestnut extract and menthol, which is a mild antiseptic that can be irritating to some skin types.

Mild Action Protection Tonic *(large size, $22):* This toner contains mostly alcohol, therefore I would not call it mild.

Re-Nutriv Gentle Skin Toner *($27.50):* Basically an alcohol-free toner that contains mostly gentle ingredients except for arnica extract. It can be irritating, but it can also have mild antiseptic benefit on the skin.

Skin Defender *(fragrance-free, $45):* This product contains a sunscreen that is not strong enough to adequately protect against the sun. It includes some typical moisturizing ingredients and a few specialty names like glycoside complex that are exclusive to this line. Other than repeating the company's description, there is no way for me to tell you what the elements really are or what they can or cannot do.

Night Repair *(fragrance-free, 1.75-ounce size, $70):* Basically a good moisturizer that contains water, thickeners and squalene (shark oil) and a handful of the latest ingredients that prevent dry skin such as proteins, cholesterol and hyaluronic acid. It won't "repair" any skin condition except for dry skin.

Eyzone *(fragrance-free, $35):* Besides the basic moisturizing ingredients like water, glycerin and butylene glycol, Eyzone also contains a few of the latest skin care ingredients that sound better than what they actually deliver in terms of wrinkles, but it will take care of dry skin.

Time Zone *($50):* The claim is that this product "reprograms skin to resist negative influences." If by negative influences they mean the drying effects of the air, this product can do that — but that's about it. The ingredients in this moisturizer are mostly water, algae extract, butylene glycol, glyceride esters (an emollient like glycerin) and squalene (shark oil). Like Eyzone and Night Repair, it also contains it's share of the latest in moisturizing ingredients.

In-Control T-Zone Solution *($16.50):* The ingredients in this product won't change your oily skin. If anything, the salicylic acid, can irritate and may cause the skin to produce even more oil.

Equalizer Oil-Free Gel *($27.50):* This gel is supposed to "monitor" and "disperse" excess oil concentration. The first ingredients are water, alcohol and phospholipids and cholesterol (both hold water to the skin). None of those ingredients can disperse or monitor oil. The phospholipids and cholesterol are good for dry skin, but the alcohol counteracts these ingredients. In my opinion, this is one confused product.

Skin Perfecting Creme *($35):* This lightweight moisturizer contains almost all of the latest fad moisturizing ingredients, plus the more typical elements to make it, if not a complicated chemical listing, a thorough one. It will take care of dry skin, and your worry that you might be missing out on a scientific miracle.

Re-Nutriv Creme *($45/$70/$135):* The main ingredients in this moisturizer are water, a form of lanolin, mineral oil and thickeners. This is a very emollient moisturizer for extremely dry skin.

Re-Nutriv Firming Eye Creme *($35):* Several state-of-the-art moisturizing ingredients are to be found in this eye cream: amino-peptide complex, serum protein, soluble collagen extract, arnica extract. These are ok, but provide more marketing than physical benefits. They simply sound good to the consumer. Arnica extract can be irritating to the skin — but it could be what temporarily firms the eye by making it slightly puffy.

Fashion Fair

Deep Cleansing Lotion *($13.50):* This is a fairly greasy cleanser that would need to be wiped off, not rinsed.

Skin Freshener I *($11):* This freshener contains mostly alcohol and is very drying, not to mention irritating, to the skin.

Skin Freshener II *($11):* This freshener has basically the same ingredients as Skin Freshener I, except in this case water is the first ingredient and alcohol the second. In the long run, you won't notice any difference, or you may find your skin becoming irritated.

Deep Pore Astringent *($12.50):* Like most astringents, this one contains mostly water, alcohol, fragrance and allantoin. You would probably be better off if it just contained water and allantoin. The fragrance and alcohol are too irritating for most all skin types.

Oil Free Moisturizer *($18.50):* This is indeed an oil-free moisturizer that contains mostly propylene glycol and thickeners. It also contains isopropyl myristate which is an ingredient believed to cause blackheads.

Eye Cream *($17.50):* This is a somewhat heavy moisturizer that contains very emollient ingredients. It will nicely take care of very dry skin, but is probably too heavy for around the eyes.

Moisturizing Lotion *($17.50):* This basic moisturizer contains water, propylene glycol, petrolatum and thickeners. It would be good for dry skin.

Moisturizing Creme *($17.50):* This is a very emollient moisturizer that would work well on extremely dry skin. It contains water, a form of lanolin, mineral oil, sesame oil, aloe vera, propylene glycol and squalene (shark oil).

La Prairie

I don't quite know how else to put this, so no beating around the bush (or the prairie). I find La Prairie one of the most overpriced skin care lines I've ever seen (although Chanel, Borghese and Yves St. Laurent aren't far behind). From what I can tell, these high-price skin care lines attract women who think that the dollars they spend provides their skin something most other women can't afford. To some extent, they're right. Those who can afford it get something other women can't: an immense amount of marketing hype and positioning. If you could read the ingredient labels and understand them, you would find their prices as ludicrous as I do. Much of La Prairie's claims are based on the use of ingredients such as placental protein, flower and herb extracts, animal collagen, and amino acids. None of the line's literature indicates that these ingredients have real positive or negative effects on the skin. Rather than refute the products' effectiveness, I suggest you compare ingredients labels. You will notice that most of the ingredients in the La Prairie products are fairly standard cosmetic ingredients. The amount of the "specialty" ingredients is almost negligible by comparison.

Essential Purifying Gel Cleanser *($45):* This cleanser contains mostly water, castor oil, propylene glycol, a liquid oil and some herb extracts. It does rinse off, but leaves a slight film behind on the skin. It also irritated the skin around my eyes.

Cellular Refining Lotion *($55):* The main ingredients in this toner are water, alcohol, propylene glycol and placental protein. No matter what the price tag and the claims about placental protein, alcohol is alcohol and can irritate the skin.

Cellular Purifying Lotion *($55):* The main ingredients in this alcohol-free toner are water, propylene glycol, liquid oils and animal protein. There are also flower and herb extracts, collagen, elastin and placental protein. It should feel good, and can help keep moisture in the skin, but this is a lot of money for flowers, herbs and animal proteins.

Emergency Tonic *($50):* This toner contains mostly water, mineral oil, alcohol, propylene glycol, placental protein and herb and flower extracts.

It also contains salicylic acid which along with the alcohol make this a fairly irritating liquid.

Cellular Skin Conditioner *($65)*: The major ingredients in this moisturizer are water, mineral oil, glycerin, thickeners and a form of lanolin. The very last ingredient is placental protein. Except for the placental protein, these are fairly typical ingredients for a good basic moisturizer. This product claims to prime the skin for all the other La Prairie treatments. I guess it depends on your definition of "prime," but there's nothing in this product that would be considered different from any other moisturizer.

Cellular Night Cream *($95)*: This is a rather rich moisturizer for dry skin that contains mineral oil, petrolatum, propylene glycol, a form of mineral oil and a form of lanolin. Again the last ingredient in the listing is placental protein.

Cellular Eye Cream *($75)*: Lighter weight than the above Cellular Night Cream, but is still very similar: water, mineral oil, thickeners, petrolatum and a form of lanolin. It also contains collagen, but we all know by now that collagen is not a miracle skin care ingredient.

Essence of Skin Caviar *($75 for 1/2 ounce)*: What would you imagine could be in a liquid that costs $2,400 a pound? The ingredients are water, propylene glycol, lactose (sugar), a form of lanolin, castor oil, panthenol (vitamin b), animal protein, glycerin and placental protein. I never thought animal protein and placental protein were worth their weight in gold! Except for the placental protein, these are fairly typical moisturizing ingredients.

Skin Caviar *($90 for 2 ounces)*: This specialty product is a lightweight oil contained in small plastic foam pellets that break open when you rub it on the skin. Cute idea. These pellets contain a form of mineral oil, water, glycerin, alcohol, an amino acid, gelatin and propylene glycol. It also contains small amounts of retinyl palmitate (vitamin A), tocopherol (vitamin A), allantoin and flower and herb extracts. It can be good for dry skin, but these ingredients just don't warrant the price tag.

Lancome

Douceur Demaquillant Nutrix *($19.50)*: This cleanser is fairly greasy, which means it needs to be wiped off. It contains mostly mineral oil, water, propylene glycol, egg oil and vegetable oil. That amount of oil would make any cleanser feel greasy.

Galatee *($19.50/$27.50):* This is supposed to be a splash-or-tissue off cleanser for all skin types. It is fairly greasy for oily or combination skin, and it doesn't really rinse off without use of a washcloth. It also contains isopropyl myristate which can cause blackheads. However, it may be good for extremely dry skin.

Ablutia Gel Moussante *(Foaming gel Cleanser, $19.50):* Most of these ingredients are found in regular shampoos. They are all fairly drying and can be irritating to the eyes and skin.

Ablutia Huile Moussante *(Foaming Oil Cleanser, $18.50):* This product is similar to the foaming gel cleanser (see above), except that the cleansing agents can be much more gentle to the skin.

Effacile *($14.50):* This is an oil-free eye makeup remover which is very gentle.

Tonique Douceur *($17.50/$26.50):* An alcohol-free toner that contains water, glycerin, sodium borate (a weak antiseptic), hexylene glycol and castor oil. This will definitely feel refreshing on dry skin. It claims to "refine" skin; if that means it can close pores, it can't.

Tonique Fraicheur *($17.50/$26):* This is very similar to the Tonique Douceur, except that it contains alcohol. You don't need the alcohol; it won't help the skin.

Controle Regulating Liquide *($18.50):* The first ingredients are water, alcohol, solvents and carbocysteine (a healing agent). The alcohol makes this lotion irritating. The claim is that it will help regulate oily skin, but this much alcohol in a product won't help regulate anything.

Noctosome Systeme *($45):* Besides having liposomes, this lightweight cream contains fairly typical moisturizing ingredients: water, macadamia oil, glycerin, vegetable oil and cholesterol. The claim is that the cream is "in harmony with skin's biological rhythms." Sounds good, but other than keeping the skin lubricated and moist, I'm not sure what rhythm it dances to.

Niosome *($35/$45):* This cream is similar to the Noctosome cream; both contain liposomes. The Niosome is slightly lighter and has a lower oil content than the Noctosome.

Oligo-Major *($37.50):* This is loaded with several of the latest scientific-sounding ingredients: serum albumin (blood from cows), a form of hyaluronic acid, spleen extract and yeast protein. It is supposed to fortify the skin. There is no evidence that any of those ingredients can feed the skin, much less "fortify" it.

Progres Eye Creme *($27.50):* This thick eye cream contains water, petrolatum, thickening agent, castor oil and shea butter. It also contains its share of fad moisturizing ingredients such as amniotic fluid, liver extract and calfskin extract. Whatever you want to believe is up to you, but I have found no evidence that these unusual ingredients have any positive or negative effects on the skin. Basically, this cream is a good emollient for dry skin around the eyes or anywhere on the face, but it won't permanently change wrinkles.

Nutribel *(Nourishing Hydrating Emulsion, $30/$45):* If you get the impression you can feed the skin from the outside in, you can't. Nevertheless, the ingredients in this lotion are good for dry skin: water, jojoba oil, glycerin, mineral oil, grapeseed oil and linoleic acid.

Bienfait Du Matin for Dry/Sensitive Skin and Normal/Oily Skin *($19.50):* There are two different types of this light cream that comes in five different colors, of which one is clear. The normal/oily formula contains mostly water, squalene (shark oil), thickeners, glycerin and kaolin (clay). The dry/sensitive formula contains water, a form of mineral oil, a form of coconut oil, talc, thickeners, glycerin and clay. Both are lightweight moisturizers, although the talc and clay can prove to be drying for some skin types. The tint in these creams is sheer to almost nonexistent. If you want to add a slight — and I mean slight — amount of all-over color that won't show a line, this one would do the trick.

Hydrix *($27.50):* This is a very rich, emollient moisturizer containing mostly water, petrolatum, mineral oil and a form of lanolin. Definitely for dry skin and those not allergic lanolin. It claims to last for 12 hours, but that wasn't my experience.

Trans-Hydrix *($28.50):* This rich cream contains water, palm oil, shea butter, black currant extract and mineral oil. I'm not sure what the black currant extract is for, but the other ingredients will help prevent dry skin. If you have extremely dry skin, the claim about lasting 24 hours is fairly exaggerated. If you do not have dry skin, then like most other rich moisturizers, it can last a while.

Cellulite "Relief" Gel *($42.50):* The only reason I'm including this is that I couldn't believe my eyes! I want to remind you that there are no creams on the market that can do anything to eliminate cellulite. I imagine that the word relief is in quotes on the packaging to obscure the meaning and to help relieve some of the pressure the FDA might put on a claim such as this.

L'Oreal

Aqua Cleansing Cream *($5 for 5 ounces):* This is more like a traditional cold cream cleanser than it is a water-soluble cream as the label suggests. It contains very rich ingredients like lanolin oil and petrolatum. It also contains clay for some reason, which you would associate more with a product designed for oily skin. Perhaps this cleanser can't make up its mind.

Active Cleansing Gel *($5 for 5 ounces):* This foaming cleanser is fairly drying. It contains somewhat strong shampoo-type detergents that can be irritating to the eyes.

Exfoliating Cream *($6):* The ingredient list reads like a basic oil-based cleanser's: water, mineral oil and thickeners. Nothing unique, but it will cleanse the face with the help of a washcloth.

Plentitude Eye Makeup Remover *($6):* This is a very gentle, non-irritating liquid.

Floral Tonic *($7.50):* This alcohol-free toner contains water, butylene glycol, salt (used as an antiseptic), an ingredient to make it pH balanced and castor oil. It can feel soothing on the skin, although the castor oil will be a problem for oily skin types.

Active Daily Moisture Oil-Free *($6.50):* This product contains water, a form of mineral oil, a form of coconut oil, glycerin and PABA. Although the product is supposed to be oil-free, two oils are present in the form of caprylic/capric/triglyceride, derived from coconut oil, and cyclomethicone. It is probably not best for someone concerned about oily skin.

Active Daily Moisturizer *($6.50):* This rich cream contains water, shea butter, vegetable oil, sesame oil, mineral oil, palm oil, and thickeners. It would be good for dry skin.

Plentitude Action Liposomes *($15.75 for 1.7 ounces):* This rich moisturizer contains water, apricot oil, a form of mineral oil, bovine extracts, glycerin, lecithin, thickeners and vegetable oil. The bovine (cow) extract has no recognized benefit to the skin, but the other ingredients, particularly the liposomes are very good.

Firming Serum Concentrate *($15.75 for 1 ounce):* This liquid contains water, hyaluronic acid, yeast protein, glycerin, spleen extract and castor oil. I wouldn't count on the yeast protein or spleen extract doing much for the skin, but the other moisturizing ingredients are good. Unfortunately, this product contains both 2-bromo-2-nitropropane and triethanolamine which together can cause skin problems.

Wrinkle Defense Cream *($10):* This product contains water, thickeners, castor oil, petrolatum, glycerin, vegetable oil, corn oil, salt, liver extract, protein and calfskin extract. The liver and calfskin extract provide no special benefits, but the other ingredients will improve dry skin.

Mary Kay

Creamy Cleanser *($9):* This creamy cleanser can't be rinsed off without the aid of a washcloth.

Deep Cleanser *($9):* This cleanser has a gentle lathering ingredient, but it also contains wax, which is not the best in a water-soluble cleanser.

Gentle Cleansing Cream *($9):* This is a traditional, greasy cold cream product containing mineral oil, water, petrolatum, beeswax, glycerin and other types of waxes. This might be gentle, but it is also quite heavy.

Gentle Action Freshener *($10):* Fairly gentle for a toner. It does contain witch hazel, but it is not one of the first five ingredients, so there is little alcohol to speak of in this product.

Blemish Control Toner *($10):* Mostly water, alcohol and propylene glycol. It also contains salicylic acid. There is no evidence that alcohol or salicylic acid will control blemishes and both ingredients are extremely irritating.

Refining Freshener *($10):* Mostly water and alcohol, which can irritate the skin.

Balancing Moisturizer *($16):* This basic moisturizer contains water, mineral oil, thickeners and propylene glycol.

Enriched Moisturizer *($16):* Not the most emollient of moisturizers for dry skin, it contains water, mineral oil, a type of mineral oil and propylene glycol.

Anti-Aging Complex *($25):* How anyone would think ingredients like water, alcohol and butylene glycol can fight aging is beyond me. This product does contain a sunscreen, although one not strong enough to keep the sun off the face, and a form of hyaluronic acid. Those are fine, but the alcohol is so drying it would negate any positive effect these moisturizing ingredients can provide. As this book went to press I learned that the ingredients of this product had been changed and the alcohol had been removed. Good move, but $25 is still a lot of money for this lightweight moisturizer.

Extra Emollient Moisturizer *($9):* This is a very rich, somewhat heavy moisturizer for dry skin that contains water, wax, squalene (shark oil), sesame oil, glycerin and soybean oil.

Oil-Control Lotion *($16):* This is another one of those "oil-free" products that contains oil derivatives with names you don't recognize as having anything to do with oil. There are no ingredients in this product that can control the amount of oil your skin produces.

Acne Treatment Gel *($16):* Contains mostly water and propylene. The active ingredient is benzyl peroxide, a popular ingredient used in dozens of products designed for acne. It is my experience that it can work in some cases, but not all, and it can, more often that not, produce skin irritation.

Neutrogena

Antiseptic Cleanser *($5.50):* This product contains a large number of ingredients that are too irritating for almost all skin types including camphor, peppermint oil, eucalyptus oil and benzethonium chloride. The recommendation on the label is too avoid the eye areas as it will burn the skin there. I would not recommend this product for any skin type.

Facial Cleansing Formula *($10):* This is a water-soluble cleanser that can tend to dry out the skin. It is milder than most, but definitely not for any one with dry skin.

Night Cream *($13 for 2.25 ounces):* This rich moisturizer contains water, glycerin, sesame oil, thickener, and petrolatum. It is good for dry skin.

Eye Cream *($8 for 1/2 ounce):* This cream contains water, a humectant, a form of coconut oil, a form of vitamin B, thickeners, mineral oil, petrolatum and hyaluronic acid. This is a good moisturizer, but not because of the vitamin B.

Neutrogena Moisture SPF 15 *($13 for 4 ounces):* This is a fairly expensive price tag for a fairly basic sunscreen. It will, however, adequately protect your face from the sun.

Oil of Olay

Olay is neither plant or animal; it is the name of a product line. For the longest time I wondered if people really thought there was some kind of oil derived from an exotic plant. Oil of Olay has several skin care products on the market and, believe it or not, some can be quite beneficial for dry skin.

Facial Cleansing Lotion *($4 for 3 ounces):* This lightweight cleanser doesn't quite rinse off without the aid of a washcloth and it can leave an oily residue on the skin.

Foaming Face Wash *($4 for 3 ounces):* This cleanser cleans the face well, without drying it out. It would be nice if it were fragrance-free like some of the other Oil of Olay products.

Water-Rinsable Cold Cream *($4.50):* This product can't rinse off with water and it leaves an oil film on the face.

Refreshing Toner *($4.50):* This toner contains alcohol, witch hazel, castor oil, aloe vera gel and allantoin. All the ingredients but the alcohol would have made this a decent toner. Alcohol and witch hazel irritate the skin and negate all the soothing benefits of the other ingredients.

Sensitive Skin Beauty Fluid *($7.25 for 4 ounces):* This lightweight fragrance-free moisturizer contains mostly water, butylene glycol, a form of mineral oil, mineral oil, thickeners, glycerin, jojoba oil, a form of vitamin E oil and castor oil. It would feel good on dry skin.

Moisture Replenishing Cream *($7.50 for 2 ounces):* This fragrance-free cream contains mostly water, mineral oil, thickeners, cholesterol, more thickeners, glycerin and castor oil. It is a good lightweight moisturizer.

Beauty Fluid *($8.50):* This is the original moisturizer that launched Oil of Olay. This pink lotion contains water, mineral oil, thickeners, cholesterol, more thickeners, castor oil and more thickeners. Not a great moisturizer, but not a bad one either. It would be good for normal to slightly dry skin.

Origins

I wanted to review the Origins' skin care system because of its clever and admirable 1990s marketing style: natural ingredients, recycled packaging (including a recycling service for the empty bottles and compacts at their counters), products that aren't tested on animals and "ancient" skin care treatments. The recycling efforts and animal-free testing are both impressive and praiseworthy examples to other cosmetics companies who continue to test their products on animals and don't use recyclable packaging. However, it's the ancient and natural stuff that I wanted the chance to investigate. Origin's basic skin care theory is presented in a very logical manner. Their assertion is that their products can "retrain" your skin to function like all skin wants to function — normally. What an enticing concept. Of course, the ingredients that supposedly retrain your skin to function normally are derived from the "ancient science of essential oils," which assumes, of course, that people from long ago had great skin because of this special knowledge. It does sound convincing, but alas there aren't any ancient people around to prove or disprove these claims. I also found the ingredient labels too ambiguous to decipher. Juxtaposed around standard skin care ingredients are "special" oils, extracts and herbs that are so obscure I couldn't find any pertinent information or the information that existed was too sparse and inadequate to utilize. With no reliable facts available, other than what the company provides (not what I would call impartial) I gave up. Even the salespeople I interviewed didn't know what many of the ingredients in their own products were. If you want to believe that herbal and flowered waters and oils can change your skin, then this is the line for you. Personally, I'm extremely skeptical and would suggest you be too.

Physicians Formula

This is one of the few cosmetics companies that publishes a list of the irritating ingredients they don't use in their products that often show up in other skin care and makeup products. None of Physicians Formula products contain things like lanolin, aluminum sulfate, benzoic acid, bovine extracts, linoleic acid, oil of walnut, salicylic acid, serum proteins or yeast extract. Even if you don't use the products, you can write to Physicians Formula Cosmetics at 230 South 9th Avenue, City of Industry, California 91746, to ask for a copy of this information. When other companies make claims that their products are hypoallergenic, you could easily use this list as a reference guide. My only issue with this skin care line is its name. It sounds as if a bunch of physicians got together and designed this line or that physicians prefer these products to others, but neither is the case. Other than that, its products are definitely worth considering.

Gentle Cleansing Lotion *($5.10/$7.20):* This cleanser is supposed to be water-soluble but it is not. It needs to be removed with the aid of a washcloth. The ingredients are water, mineral oil, petrolatum and thickeners. It's actually a better moisturizer than it is a cleanser.

Gentle Cleansing Cream *($4.85/$5.40):* This cleanser is like a traditional cold cream, containing mostly mineral oil, water, petrolatum and beeswax.

Deep Cleanser *($4.35/$6.40):* Like so many cleansers recommended for oily or combination skin, this one contains ingredients that are similar to shampoo and can irritate both the skin and the eyes.

Deep Pore Cleansing Gel *($5.40):* This cleanser is almost identical to the Deep Cleanser. It is very similar to a shampoo and can be drying and irritating for almost all skin types.

Eye Makeup Remover Lotion *($5.10):* This is very similar to the Gentle Cleansing Lotion with only minor differences. You don't need both. The Gentle Cleansing Lotion will take off eye makeup as well as the face makeup.

Gentle Refreshing Toner *($4.35/$6.40):* This alcohol-free toner contains mostly water and glycerin. It also contains a small quantity of hyaluronic acid. It should feel very soothing on most skin types.

Vital Defense Moisture Lotion *($6.90):* This is a good basic oil-free sunscreen with an SPF of 15. Keep in mind that oil-free doesn't mean that the wax-like thickeners in the cream won't make you breakout.

Emollient Oil *($5.50):* This feels great on dry skin. It is a very thick, velvety oil containing safflower oil, sesame oil, petrolatum and a form of lanolin.

Oil-Control Moisturizer *($5.40):* Like most oil-free moisturizers this product contains mostly water, thickeners and some emollients. It also contains bentonite, a white clay, that can absorb oil to some degree, but the clay can also absorb some of the water and emollients in the product itself. How much the product can "control" oily skin is questionable.

Sun Products: For price and reliable ingredients, I would encourage trying any of the Physicians Formula sun products.

Pond's

Water Rinsable Cleanser *($4.50):* I am always looking for inexpensive, quality water-soluble cleansers. When I saw the ad for this cleanser I was intrigued. Unfortunately there is nothing water-soluble about this product. The main ingredients are water, mineral oil and beeswax. If anything, the cleanser leaves an oily film on the skin.

Water Rinsable Cleanser for Sensitive Skin *($4.50):* This cleanser is almost identical to the one above, which means it isn't what I would call water-soluble.

Facial Cleansing Foam *($4.50):* This would actually be a good gentle water-soluble cleanser if it didn't also include mineral oil, beeswax and ceresin, all of which can leave an oily film on the face.

Extra Rich Moisturizer *($4.50 for 3.9 ounces):* This is a fairly basic moisturizer that contains water, mineral oil, emollient, petrolatum, glycerin and thickeners. It can be quite good for dry skin.

Prescriptives

Prescriptives is one of the only department store cosmetics lines to be entirely fragrance-free. That is a praiseworthy effort in a sea of competitive products that rely on smell more than quality to sell products. That's not to say I find the rest of Prescriptives formulations or prices equally exceptional, but the omission of fragrance is a healthy step in the right direction.

Line Preventor *($45):* The first ingredients in this product won't do anything to prevent lines on the face. The product is basically water, a humectant, thickener, butylene glycol, glycerin and a mineral-type oil. There is a sunscreen in this product, but it is not strong enough to adequately protect the skin from the sun.

Extra Firm Skin Care Concentrate *($55):* The basic ingredients are fairly typical for a moisturizer. The ingredient that is supposed to convince you that the lotion will firm the skin is the tissue extract. There is no evidence that tissue extract can affect the skin one way or the other. Otherwise, it is a good moisturizer.

Simply Moisture *($35):* This product contains a sunscreen, but the SPF is under 15. It is otherwise a good basic, lightweight moisturizer that contains water, butylene glycol, glycerin, several different forms of protein, and several other popular skin care ingredients like hyaluronic acid, retinyl palmitate, herbs and oil. The creamy aspect of the protein is more beneficial to the skin than the protein itself.

Multi-Moisture Pure Hydrating Cream *($37.50):* This product also contains a low-rated sunscreen and, although a cream not a lotion, is essentially identical to the Simply Moisture. It is a good basic skin cream.

Eyewear *($35):* This is a good moisturizer that consists primarily of water, butylene glycol, tissue matrix extract, mineral oil and squalene (shark oil). The tissue matrix extract sounds good, but I wasn't able to find out where the tissue is from or what it is, so your guess is as good as mine.

Revlon (Drugstore and Department Store)

Clean & Clear Facial Cleansing Gel *($2.75 for 8 ounces):* I like this cleanser quite a bit. It cleans the skin without drying it out and removes all makeup, including the eye makeup. I would prefer it didn't contain any coloring agents like their sensitive skin formula does, but still it should feel quite good on most skin types.

Clean & Clear Facial Cleansing Gel for Sensitive Skin *($2.75 for 8 ounces):* I also like this cleanser quite a bit. It removes all the makeup and doesn't burn the eyes. It should feel excellent on normal to dry skin.

Clean & Clear Skin Cleansing Lotion *($2.75 for 8 ounces):* This is an extremely irritating toner that contains alcohol, water, benzoic acid (a preservative), camphor, eucalyptus oil and peppermint oil.

Clean & Clear Astringent Cleansing Lotion *($2.75):* Almost identical to the Clean & Clear Cleansing Lotion, this astringent is extremely irritating and can be harmful to the skin.

Clean & Clear Facial Cleansing Liquid, Unscented *($3.50):* This cleanser is more like shampoo than it is like a facial cleanser. It can be drying to the skin.

Clean & Clear Moisture Firm Facial Treatment *($4.85):* This is a very good, lightweight moisturizer that contains water, thickener, propylene glycol, butylene glycol, thickener, chitin extract (a soothing agent) and hyaluronic acid.

Clean & Clear Sensitive Skin Moisture Lotion *($2.75 for 4 ounces):* This lightweight moisturizer contains water, butylene glycol, thickener, mineral oil, propylene glycol and more thickeners. It would be ok for normal skin, but it won't do much for dry skin.

Clean & Clear Oil-Free Facial Moisture Lotion *($2.75 for 4 ounces):* This is one of the few oil-free moisturizers that is truly oil-free. All it contains is water, an agent to help water penetrate the skin, propylene glycol and thickeners. It probably won't do much for dry or normal skin and it probably isn't necessary for someone with oily skin, but it is indeed an oil-free moisturizer.

European Collagen Complex Cream *($13.95 for 3 ounces):* This is a fairly rich moisturizer for dry skin that contains water, thickener, propylene glycol, collagen, sweet almond oil, thickeners, mineral oil, more thickeners, olive oil, lecithin and lanolin oil.

European Collagen Complex Lotion *($9.50 for 4 ounces):* This lightweight lotion contains water mineral oil, propylene glycol, collagen, thickeners, clay, lecithin, petrolatum and talc. I would say that this is a good moisturizer if it weren't for the talc and clay. Those two ingredients would absorb moisture from the skin.

Eterna 27 Gentle Cleansing Cream *($11.50):* This is a traditional wipe-off cold cream product.

Eterna 27 Gentle Cleansing Lotion *($11.50):* This is a lighter weight cleanser than the one above, but one still too greasy to rinse off easily without the aid of a washcloth.

Eterna 27 Gentle Toning Lotion *($11.50):* I wouldn't call this toner gentle at all. It contains witch hazel, menthol and benzethonium chloride. All are fairly irritating to the skin.

Eterna 27 All Day Moisture Lotion *($12.50 for 2 ounces):* This is a very emollient, good moisturizer for dry skin that contains water, propylene glycol, thickener, olive oil, a form of lanolin, thickener, squalene (shark oil) and protein.

Eterna 27 All Day Moisture Cream *($12.50):* This cream is very similar to the lotion above. The major difference is that it contains more thickeners. It would be good for dry skin.

Eterna 27 with Exclusive Progenitin *($26 for 4 ounces):* Now I know this is going to sound strange, so remember I'm only describing this product, I didn't formulate it. The active ingredient in this product is called pregnenolone acetate. It is derived from the urine of pregnant women and is considered to be an anti-inflammatory (cortizone) agent. Therefore, this moisturizer is actually a very mild topical cortizone-type cream. In my opinion, unless your dry skin is a result of a dermatitis this cream is unnecessary. Plus there are cheaper topical cortizone creams on the market. Beyond the price, this is a very emollient cream for dry skin only that contains water, mineral oil, beeswax, petrolatum, propylene glycol, thickener, almond oil, avocado oil and sesame oil. Although, if you have a tendency to breakout, you would not want to use this product.

Shiseido

Facial Cleansing Foam *(for oily skin $20):* This is a fairly traditional foaming cleanser that contains gentle detergent agents. It is a good cleanser, but it can leave the face feeling somewhat dry.

Facial Cleansing Foam Concentrate *(for dry skin $27):* This cleanser is almost identical to the one above, except that this one contains a small amount of hyaluronic acid, which won't help counter the drying effect it can have on the face.

Gel Action Makeup Remover *($22):* This cleanser is somewhat unique because it contains neither oils, detergent cleansing agents or soap. It is indeed gentle on the skin and a good cleanser.

Facial Cleansing Cream *($22):* This product is a fairly typical cold cream that needs to be wiped off. It contains mineral oil, water, squalene, thickener, propylene glycol, petrolatum and tallow.

Washing Grains *($22):* Bascially this product contains cleansing ingredients that are found in soaps and shampoos. It can leave the skin feeling dry.

Facial Astringent Lotion *($20):* Like most astringents this product contains mostly water and alcohol and is too irritating for most skin types.

Facial Softening Lotion *($33):* This is a toner that is mostly water, propylene glycol and alcohol. Alcohol is never great for the skin.

Facial Soothing Lotion *($26.50):* This lotion is designed for oily skin and it can indeed absorb oil, but I would not necessarily call it soothing. The ingredients are water, butylene glycol and two types of clay.

Facial Moisturizing Concentrate Lotion *($34):* This is a good moisturizer for dry skin that contains mostly water, squalene (shark oil), glycerin, petrolatum and propylene glycol.

Eye Wrinkle Cream Concentrate *($40):* This very rich, thick cream contains mostly water, squalene (shark oil), mineral oil, petrolatum and sodium pca. It won't change the wrinkles around your eye, but it will improve your dry skin.

Bio Performance Super Revitalize Creme *($60):* The brochure for this product in of itself was amazing. A four-page, full-color glossy brochure, including graphs and charts, explained of why this product would do more for your skin "than ever dreamed possible." Despite this presentation, it is a good lightweight moisturizer that is predominantly water and glycerin. It also contains all of the latest moisturizing ingredients, but nothing more.

Bio Performance Synchro Serum *($75):* The brochure for this product is impressive. If you can interpret the information, you must have a degree in chemistry. The before and after pictures, although convincing, are misleading. There is no explanation as to what shape the "before" skin was in prior to using this product. There are two vials in this package that you're supposed to combine. The Essence contains water, glycerin, butylene glycol, alcohol, a humectant and lecithin. The Powder contains a thickener, a protein, an amino acid, hyaluronic acid and sodium pca. Mixed together, these two compounds do make a good moisturizer, but nothing more.

UV Facial Protection Complex *($20):* This lotion only has an SPF of 8 which is not enought to adequately protect the face from the sun.

B.H-24 *($65 for a total of 2 ounces):* There are two very small bottles of liquid in this product that are supposed to be worn under your regular moisturizer. The Day Essence contains mostly water, butylene glycol, glycerin and alcohol. It also contains smaller amounts of collagen, hyaluronic acid and chondroitin. The Night Essence essentially has the same formulation. This product is basically an overpriced toner. I always have a problem with products that are marketed as adding moisture to the skin, but the product contains alcohol, which dries out the skin.

Ultima II

The Cleanser *($13.50):* Like many water-soluble cleansers, this cleanser contains a gentle shampoo detergent called sodium laureth sulfate. It may be drying for normal and dry skin types.

Extraordinary Lotion Cleanser *($17):* This cleanser does not rinse off without the help of a washcloth.

CHR Extraordinary Gentle Clarifier *($17):* This alcohol-free toner would be good for dry skin. The main ingredients are water, propylene glycol, a form of lanolin, collagen and protein.

Pro Collagen Face and Throat Cream *($40):* The first ingredients are water, a form of mineral oil, propylene glycol, butylene glycol, collagen and mineral oil. This moisturizer would be good for dry skin.

Moisture Lotion Concentrate *($28):* This product contains mostly water, propylene glycol, a form of lanolin, thickeners and collagen. It would be good for dry skin.

The Moisturizer *($20):* This is very similar to the Moisture Lotion Concentrate and would be good for dry skin.

Photo-Aging Shield *($36):* This is not a good sunscreen because the SPF is under 15. It also contains alcohol which can dry and irritate the skin.

Pro Collagen *($40):* This moisturizer does contain collagen but not much else. It would be a good moisturizer for normal skin, but dry skin may need more emollients than this one has.

Mineral Mask *($15):* Along with the minerals you get in this mask, you'll also find alcohol, which will irritate and dry out the skin.

Victoria Jackson

There are five products in the Victoria Jackson skin care line that are supposed to be suitable for all skin types. It's an interesting and unusual concept for a cosmetics company and one that I find hard to accept. Skin care for someone with oily skin cannot be the same for someone with extremely dry or normal skin. Still, I like some of these products very much and the price range (if you buy more than $20 worth of products at a time) is quite reasonable.

Note: *The first price listed is for the individual product; the second price applies when you order more than $20 worth of products at one time.*

Facial Cleanser *($12.50/$7.25):* You are meant to wipe-off your makeup using this watery cleanser applied to a cotton ball and then rinse off any residue. The main ingredients are water, a form of coconut oil (that is considered to be a good, non-greasy cleansing agent), collagen, hyaluronic acid and sodium pca. It actually feels quite light on the skin, and the ingredients are very moisturizing, but I'm still not a proponent of wiping off makeup.

Toning Mist *($13.50/$7.75):* This alcohol-free toner contains water, aloe vera gel, sodium pca, hyaluronic acid, collagen and panthenol. It feels good and the ingredients can keep moisture in the skin without leaving a hint of oily residue. It would be better, however, if this product didn't contain fragrance.

Moisturizer *($19.50/$11.75):* This product contains mostly water, a form of mineral oil, propylene glycol, thickener and castor oil. It also contains collagen, hyaluronic acid, tocopherol, and retinyl palmitate. This is a good lightweight moisturizer.

Eye Repair Gel *($18.50/$10.50 for 1/2 ounce):* This gel contains water, propylene glycol, sodium pca, collagen, hyaluronic acid and panthenol. It is actually very similar to the Toning Mist, only ten times more expensive by weight.

Firming Gel Masque *($16.50/$9.95):* This mask contains water, an ingredient that allows the product to harden on the face, along with aloe vera gel, collagen, hyaluronic acid, sodium pca, collagen, panthenol and glycerin. Again, this product is much like the Toning Mist except for the ingredient that makes turns the liquid into a gel, which can be irritating to the skin.

UNDERSTANDING THE INGREDIENTS

The following is a list of the ingredients I've talked about throughout this entire chapter and in several other sections of the book. You will also notice that many of them are listed on the label of the skin care products you are presently using. Each ingredient is examined briefly as to what it is and what it can or cannot do for the skin. Although there are many claims about skin care formulations that don't make sense and many that you could easily do without, there are many that are beneficial to the skin. The information included here is truly the nuts and bolts of the cosmetics industry. Understanding the ingredient label may not change the way you buy skin care products altogether, but it will definitely make you more aware of what you're buying.

Acetone: This is used in some astringents and toners for its ability to remove oil from the skin. It is extremely drying and can cause severe irritation.

Alcohol, SD Alcohol 10-40: Alcohol is found in many different types of skin care products, but most frequently in astringents, toners and fresheners. It can severely dry out the skin and the resulting dryness can irritate the skin.

Algae Extract: Derived from seaweed and any water where green stuff grows. The claim is that it can do something special for wrinkles; it can't.

Allantoin: This cosmetic ingredient is well known, legitimately, for its ability to help heal and soothe the skin.

Amino Acids, Proteins and Animal Protein: Amino acids constitute the protein in human skin. Twenty-two of these extremely complex substances are used in cosmetics. Proteins provide a smooth covering on the skin and they are considered to be beneficial in helping the skin absorb water. They provide no other benefit such as building or supplementing the protein in your own skin.

Ammonium Glycerhizinate: This strange sounding ingredient is a very good anti-inflamatory agent. It helps soothe skin and reduce irritation.

Amniotic Fluid: The liquid surrounding the embryo in animals is where this ingredient comes from. In cosmetics the claim is that this fluid can rejuvenate the skin. There are no independent studies that support this claim.

Animal Thymus Extract, Animal Tissue Extract: This is the tissue from either the thymus, testes, ovaries, udder and placenta of a cow or pig. The claim is that this stuff can change the wrinkles on your face. None of it can change a wrinkle anywhere on your body.

2-Bromo-2-Nitropane-1, 3 Diol: When this ingredient and the compound Triethanolamine are used together in a cosmetic they can combine to form a potential carcinogenic material.

Camphor: This can cause irritation upon contact with the skin.

Caprylic/Capric/Lauric Triglycerides: This is an oily substance derived from coconut oil and it helps keep water in the skin.

Cholesterol, Triglycerides, Phospholipids, Lecithin: These elements are all found in human tissue. In cosmetics, they very nicely help bind water to the skin and keep it there. Nothing special, but very good for dry skin.

Collagen and Elastin: These two well known ingredients keep water in the skin. The distorted belief that somehow collagen and elastin rubbed on the skin would help rebuild the collagen and elastin in your own skin is hopefully a thing of the past. The collagen and elastin found in cosmetics, because of its structure cannot even penetrate the skin.

Fatty Acids: Stearic acid is the most popular fatty acid you will find used in cosmetics. It is a substance found in skin tissue. Used in a cosmetic, it helps keep water in the skin.

Glycerin: This is a fairly standard skin care ingredient that helps attract water to the skin and keep it moist.

Hyaluronic Acid: You will be hearing quite a bit about hyaluronic acid over the next several years. It will be one of the buzzwords of the 1990s, just as collagen and elastin were in the 1980s. Hyaluronic acid is a mucopolysaccharide (another ingredient you will find in skin care products), which is a basic element found in skin tissue. When used in creams and lotions it helps water penetrate the skin. There is no evidence that hyaluronic acid can aid the skin besides keeping the surface soft.

Isopropyl Myristate: This chemical has a reputation for causing blackheads and other skin irritations when used in high concentrations of 10 percent or greater. Most cosmetics don't use that much, but you would not want to find this in the first few ingredients in a cosmetic you were thinking of using.

Kaolin, Bentonite: Both are clays that are used in cosmetics to aid in the absorption of excess oil. They can be slightly irritating.

Lanolin: The only negative thing you can say about lanolin is that it is a potential skin sensitizer. Other than that, it is very effective at keeping the skin moist and supple. You will see several types of lanolin on skin care product labels: hydroxylated lanolin, lanolin alcohols, lanolin oil and acetylated lanolin. All of these work as well or better than pure lanolin in helping keep moisture in the skin.

Liposomes: Liposomes are an interesting, unique chemical compound. You will see more and more of it used in skin care products because of the way it helps keep water and oil in the skin for longer periods of time than other skin care ingredients can.

Minerals: Minerals such as salt (sodium chloride), iodine, magnesium, chloride and potassium are potential skin irritants when used in cosmetics.

Mineral Oil: For some reason, this widely used cosmetic ingredient has gained a bad reputation in the past. In spite of the occasional bad press, mineral oil is considered to be one of the most non-irritating cosmetic ingredients available and is superior at keeping water in the skin.

Mucopolysaccharides, Glycosamnioglycans: Along with collagen and elastin, these substances are found in the lower layers of human skin. In skin care products they offer exactly the same benefit to the skin as collagen and elastin.

Neural Lipid Extract, Epidermal Lipid Extract: This is the fat tissue from the skin and brain of animals. The cosmetics industry would like you to believe that they have some rejuvenating effects on the skin. There is no evidence that these extracts can do anything for the skin, much less make it look younger.

Oil: Oils keep water in the skin. There are lots of oils used in skin care products, everything from jojoba oil to egg oil, rice bran oil, castor oil, and shark oil (squalene), and the list goes on and on. You would not want to buy a moisturizer, and you probably wouldn't be able to find one, that didn't use a combination of oils as the primary ingredients.

Petrolatum: Petrolatum is one of the more effective moisturizing ingredients around. Study after study indicates it performs as well or better than any other skin care ingredient for keeping water in the skin.

Propylene Glycol, Butylene Glycol and Polyethylene Glycol (PEG): These skin care basics are present in almost every cleanser, toner, lotion, cream or specialty product you will ever buy. These ingredients help attract moisture to the skin and help the product spread evenly over the skin.

Salicylic Acid: This ingredient can be very irritating to the skin. It is used frequently in acne preparations for its ability to exfoliate the skin.

Serum Albumin, Serum Protein: These elements are derived from the blood of cows or pigs and are used as moisturizing ingredients. Neither provide any benefit for the skin in spite of their sounding like a blood transfusion.

Sodium Lauryl Sulfate, Zinc Lauryl Sulfate, Ammonium Lauryl Sulfate, and Magnesium Lauryl Sulfate: These compounds are all cleansing agents found mostly in shampoos and skin cleansers. These are considered to be very drying when used as the primary ingredient in a skin cleanser.

Sodium Laureth Sulfate, Magnesium Laureth Sulfate: Both of these, and a dozen or so similar sounding ingredients, are considered to be more gentle detergent cleansing agents than the ones listed above. They are found most often in shampoos and water-soluble cleansers. They can be gentle, but they can also be somewhat drying on the skin.

Sodium PCA: This ingredient is a component of human skin that is used in cosmetics for its ability to hold water to the skin.

Spleen Extract: (See Animal Thymus Extract)

Tissue Matrix Extract: (See Animal Thymus Extract)

Tocopherol: This is the chemical name for vitamin E. It is used in cosmetics as an anti-oxidant, which means it helps keep the air off the face and that helps prevent dehydration. Vitamins do not feed the skin in any way from the outside in.

Vitamin A, Retinyl Palmitate and Retinol: These ingredients are frequently found in cosmetics nowadays. Retinol and retinyl palmitate are derivatives of vitamin A. Vitamin A is also the source for the prescription drug Retin-A. This association with Retin-A misleads many consumers into believing that products containing these ingredients can provide the same or similar benefits to the skin as Retin-A can. None of the claims is true. Even if it were true, you would not want to use a cosmetic that could have the same effects on the skin as Retin-A. Retin-A is quite potent and can change the skin. When something is strong enough to actually change the structure of skin, believe me there are going to be some potential negative side effects. For the most part vitamin A, retinyl palmitate and retinol are fairly benign on the skin. They may have some benefits in terms of allowing moisture to penetrate the skin but that's about it.

Water: Dry skin or mature skin contains an increased number of dried-out skin cells. Water rehydrates these cells. Whether it is fancy water from the Swiss Alps or natural spring water, demineralized water or water extracted from plants or flowers, water is water and it is what you need to have on the face, or in your skin care product, if a moisturizer is going to have any effect on your face.

Witch Hazel: This compound is comprised of about 15 – 20% alcohol. It is considered to be a mild skin irritant. Many products that claim they are alcohol-free often contain witch hazel.

Overheard comment from a woman buying makeup:

"It's probably still true that it is better for a woman to have beauty than brains because men see better than they think."

CHAPTER EIGHT

The Products
You and I Liked the Most

SURVEY RESPONSE

When I decided to write this book, I began by designing a questionnaire to evaluate how women felt about the makeup they were already using. The survey was mailed to over 500 women. Over 300 responded. The answers and comments were enlightening. The information helped me understand what women did and did not want from the cosmetics they were using. It also guided me in my choice of which cosmetics lines I reviewed.

As helpful as this data was, there were times I definitely didn't agree with the product critiques I received. Many women liked eyeshadows and blushes from various lines that I would consider too shiny to wear. When a woman complained that her blush didn't last, there was no way for me to tell what was causing the problem. If someone wearing blush tends to rub her face during the day or if her work entails a lot of phone calling, the blush might not be the problem. Or if an eyeshadow was assessed as being difficult to put on, I couldn't tell if that was due to the product itself or the woman's application technique. Without more specific information, some of the answers were interesting but not constructive. Most of the time, however, the critiques of the various products were a great resource to consider in my own evaluations and it made my job easier. Many women were eager to tell me which products caused them allergic reactions. For the most part, I didn't use those comments, unless there was a large number of similar experiences. What makes one person's skin react, may not effect another person.

The following is a summary (alphabetized by company) of the most typical responses from the survey:

Alexandra de Markoff's 86-1/2 foundation feels like it is just laying on my pores.

There must be somebody other than Alexandra de Markoff who makes an eyeshadow like "Pinked," because I refuse to pay $25 for a single eyeshadow. There is a limit!

Almay's undereye concealer goes on easily and covers well by just using a little bit.

I love Almay's One Coat Mascara and Mascara Plus.

Almay's pressed powder for oily skin is good for touch-ups.

I love Alpha Keri Body Lotion.

Borghese's eyeshadows crease on me, even with their shadow base.

I like Chanel's eyeshadows, but the price is crazy. They don't seem any different than Lancome's which cost a lot less.

Chanel's Teint Pur foundation goes on sheer, yet covers well.

Chanel's powder blush has nice colors but they seem to fade quickly.

Chanel's waterproof mascara clumps.

Chanel's Sheer Brilliance lipstick feathers into the lines around my mouth, but the colors are beautiful.

Charles of the Ritz makes the only eyeliner that stays on me.

Christian Dior's Teint d'Ete was supposed to be light and sheer; it went on well, but it also looked fake and dark.

Christian Dior's foundations look pasty on my very white skin.

Christian Dior makes a great mascara.

The best pressed powder I've found is Christian Dior's!

Cover Girl's foundation colors are always too pink or too peach for my skin tone.

Cover Girl's Translucent Medium powder has a great color and it lasts.

Cover Girl's Continuous Coverage lipstick really lasts!

Clinique's liquid eyeliner is good and doesn't smear, but it runs out too fast.

I like Clinique's Balanced Foundation. It goes on light and looks natural.

Clinique's Advanced Concealer has good matte coverage but too much will cake and look thick.

I love Clinique's lipsticks!

Clinique's lipsticks don't last.

Clinique's Stay True foundation was too heavy and thick feeling for me.

Clinique's Pore Minimizer doesn't last and is hard to put on.

Elizabeth Arden's Mousse Foundation looks great and the coverage is good. Plus the last time I checked, it wasn't that expensive.

Elizabeth Arden's Mousse concealer is useless and too much comes out all at once.

Elizabeth Arden's Matte Finish foundation feels wonderful and lasts.

Estee Lauder's Polished Performance foundation goes on well, feels good and provides light coverage.

I have about seven shades of Estee Lauder lipsticks and they are all soft and have good staying power.

Fashion Fair's Perfect Finish Oil-Free, Fragrance-Free foundation is smooth and my exact skin color.

I love Lancome's products, particularly the cream-to-powder blushes, eye pencils and mascaras, but they are just too expensive.

I used to work for Lancome. They have a mascara called Keracils. We had so many returned, you wouldn't believe it. Lancome finally had to reformulate!

I have several Lancome lipsticks and they are great!

I like L'Oreal's Mattique foundation very much. The coverage is good and it lasts all day.

L'Oreal's Lashout is one of the best mascaras I've ever used.

L'Oreal's Micro Blush is not only inexpensive, it goes on smooth and soft.

L'Oreal's lipsticks have beautiful colors and creamy consistency.

L'Oreal's Le Grand Kohl eye pencil seem as good as any I've tried at the department store.

Maybelline's Great Lash Mascara is fabulous!

Maybelline's Ultra-lash Mascara clumped and flaked all over the place.

Maybelline's Long Lasting lipstick changed color on my lips.

Maybelline's Turning Point eyeliner and eyebrow pencil lasts long, goes on smoothly and is very inexpensive.

Max Factor's Erase Line Filler and Coty Overnight Success Instant Face Smoother didn't work for me. Both became dry and flaky after they dried.

Max Factor's New Definition lipstick was too dry and matte, but it lasted all day.

Max Factor's 2000 Calorie Mascara doesn't flake and lasts all day.

Physicians Formula foundations contain a SPF of 15, which is great because I don't need to wear a separate moisturizer that contains a sunscreen at the same time.

Prescriptives' Makeup 1 is a great foundation and a great color match for my skin!

Prescriptives' Yellow/Orange eyeshadow set looked great in the container, but didn't apply well. It took a lot of powder to show any color.

Prescriptives' lipstick, lipliner and eyeliner are excellent products, but very expensive.

I sometimes think I shouldn't like Revlon's blushes as much as I do, because they're so inexpensive. But I do; they're great.

I like Shiseido lipsticks; they are creamy and feel great on.

Just because products are called pure doesn't mean you won't be allergic to them. I found this out the hard way.

Why are there clear mascaras? Kind of like the Emperor's New Clothes.

I hate the excessive packaging!

Most translucent powders look ashy on black skin.

THE PRODUCTS YOU LIKED THE MOST

After reading through each survey the overall positive responses were compiled for each product category. The results are as follows:

Foundation: All of Lancome's foundations were rated as being superior. The only foundation of Lancome's that received negative comments was their oil-free Maquicontrole. Second in popularity to Lancome's foundations was Clinique's, although Clinique's Pore Minimizer also received poor comments. The only oil-free foundation to be praised consistently was Mary Kay's and Estee Lauder's.

Concealer: There was no winner in this category. Women either didn't use it or they didn't like the one they were using.

Blush: Clinique, Estee Lauder, Mary Kay and Lancome received the most positive comments. Maybelline was rated positively most of the time; except the occasional comments that mentioned the colors went on too soft and sheer.

Eyeshadow: Maybelline, Estee Lauder, Mary Kay, Revlon, Cover Girl and Clinique were all listed as favorites. (Most women didn't complain about shiny eyeshadows, so take this summary cautiously.)

Lipstick: Lancome, Clinique, Estee Lauder, Cover Girl, Revlon, Mary Kay and Almay were rated the highest. All the comments indicated that these lipsticks went on well, lasted, and felt creamy, not greasy.

Eye and Brow Pencils: Cover Girl, Maybelline, Lancome, Clinique and Revlon all received high marks for their various types of pencils.

Lip Pencil: Lancome and Clinique got the most positive responses in this category, but otherwise women did not feel strongly about the lip pencils they were using.

Mascara: Maybelline (Great Lash), Lancome, L'Oreal (Lash Out) and Estee Lauder were the leaders in this area.

THE PRODUCTS I LIKED THE MOST

The recommendations below reflect summaries of the individual reviews in Chapter Six and Seven. Be sure to read over the more detailed product evaluations in that chapter before making any decisions. There are a handful of products listed below from companies I did not review in the previous chapters. I've included these products because they worked so well. I hope all these recommendations will make shopping for makeup a more stress-free experience.

Foundation: There are many wonderful foundations on the market at both the department store and drugstore. In spite of that, I don't encourage women to shop at the drugstore for foundations. Foundations need to match the skin exactly and, because you must also be comfortable with the coverage, you need to try the product on before you buy it. Only L'Oreal consistently has testers for every foundation shade, but many of their colors are too peach or rose to recommend. Max Factor's Satin Splendor (cream-to-powder) foundation is great and the colors very reliable. The same is true for Revlon's Powder Cream Makeup Base and their Springwater Oil-Free Makeup, but again you have to guess which color is best for you and that can be a problem. You don't need to spend a lot of money on foundation, but the department store lines are really your best option.

For general excellence, high marks go to Lancome, Clinique, Borghese, Fashion Fair, Ultima II's New Nakeds, Prescriptives (not including their Oil-Free Foundation that is half glycerin and half talc), Shiseido (but not their Dual Compact Powder), Origins, Mary Kay, Charles of the Ritz (but be careful; some of the foundation shades are quite pink and peach) and Estee Lauder. I am very fond of Borghese's Liquid Powder Makeup, but it only works on normal or slightly combination skin types. For best buys I would strongly encourage Clinique, Fashion Fair, Ultima II's New Nakeds, Mary Kay (see warning concerning these foundations in Chapter Six) and Charles of the Ritz (which has great foundations, but some of the colors are not the best).

For oily skin, my favorite foundations are Clinique's Stay True

Makeup, Prescriptives' 100% Oil-Free Liquid Makeup, Ultima II's New Nakeds Oil-Control Foundation, Fashion Fair's Oil-Free Liquid Foundation, Mary Kay's Oil-Free Foundation, Lancome's Maquicontrole (provides heavy, but long-lasting, shine-free coverage), L'Oreal's Mattique, Revlon's Springwater Oil-Free Foundation and Estee Lauder's Demi Matte. Elizabeth Arden's Simply Mousse Makeup is worth checking out, even though the mousse-style container can be tricky to use. Definitely the best buys in oil-free foundations are by Revlon (although there are no testers available), Lancome, L'Oreal, Clinique, Fashion Fair and Ultima II.

For normal skin, and some combination skin types, I simply love almost all the cream-to-powder foundations I've tried on the market. Revlon's Powder Cream and Max Factor's Satin Splendor are excellent and very inexpensive. Higher priced and equally wonderful are Adrien Arpel's Creme Powder Foundation, Borghese's Liquid Powder Makeup, Lancome's Creme Compact Makeup, Shiseido's Creme Powder Compact and Ultima II's Brush-On Foundation. The best buys without sacrificing quality are by Revlon, Max Factor and Ultima II.

Note: *Borghese's Liquid Powder Makeup is very expensive, but it happens to be very good as well as unique. It is a liquid that comes in a compact, goes on slightly damp and then dries to a powder. For those with normal skin and extra money, this is a foundation worth checking out.*

There are a wide variety of liquid and compact foundations available for dry skin. My only warning is to be careful choosing a foundation that is too heavy and greasy. Having dry skin does not mean your skin needs to be greased up. Be careful! The best foundations for dry skin are Borghese's Milano 2000 and Lumina Compact Foundation (both are excellent, although the Milano 2000 is highly fragranced), Clinique's Balanced Makeup and Extra Help, Estee Lauder's Country Mist and Polished Performance (though Polished Performance is my preference), Fashion Fair's Liquid Sheer Foundation, Lancome's Maquivelour, Mary Kay's Formula 2 (see warning concerning these foundations in Chapter Six), Prescriptives' Makeup 1 and Makeup 2 (though my preference is Makeup 1) and Shiseido's Stick Foundation.

As I said before, there are a few good, very inexpensive foundations at the drugstore, but since you can't try most of them on before you buy, you're better off at the department store. Having said that, the "best buys" for all skin types are made by Clinique, Fashion Fair, Mary Kay and Ultima II. The money-saving drugstore products that you are least likely to make mistakes with are L'Oreal's Mattique, Revlon's Springwater

Makeup and Powder Creme, and Max Factor's Satin Splendor.

Concealer: Trying to find a good undereye concealer is not an easy task at the cosmetics counters. Many were either too greasy, too dry, too thick, too peach, too pink, too dark or too expensive. Surprisingly enough, the best undereye concealers I found were at the drugstore — isn't that a relief. The concealers I tried at the cosmetic counters were, for the most part, fairly good, but given the excellent assortment I found at the drugstores, why bother! The best concealers are Almay's Cover-Up Stick and Undereye Cover Cream, The Body Shop's Concealer Sticks, Cover Girl's Moisture Wear Concealer, Clinique's Quick Corrector, Fashion Fair's Fragrance-Free Cover Stick and Regular Coverstick, Mary Kay's Touch-On Concealer, Max Factor's Erase, Maybelline's Shine-Free Cover Stick, Origin's (the light shade only), Prescriptives' Camouflage Cream and Revlon's (drugstore) New Complexion Concealer.

The best buys are made by Almay, The Body Shop, Cover Girl, Fashion Fair, Max Factor, Maybelline and Revlon.

Finishing Powder: I don't think it makes sense to spend too much money on a finishing powder because there is so little difference between products. More then 95 percent of them are talc-based; the rest of the ingredients vary only slightly. When I think of the number of pressed powders priced between $16 and $30, I just shake my head at the audacity of the cosmetics companies. Unfortunately, it is hard to recommend with any enthusiasm the finishing powders available at the drugstore. Some of these are superior products, but there is no way to test the color. For drugstore finishing powders I will make my suggestions based on what I think are the safest choices, but if you are inexperienced, trying on a powder is generally the best way to make a decision.

The best finishing powders are Almay's Shine Free and Sheer Finish, Borghese's (both loose and pressed), Charles of the Ritz's Ready Blended Pressed Powders, Clinique's (both loose and pressed), Elizabeth Arden's Flawless Finish Pressed Powder, Fashion Fair's (both loose and pressed), Lancome's (loose and pressed), L'Oreal's (pressed only), Mary Kay's (pressed only), Maybelline's (pressed only), Prescriptives' (loose and pressed), Revlon's Springwater Powder Oil-Free, Shiseido's (pressed only), Ultima II's (pressed only) and Victoria Jackson's. The best buys without sacrificing quality are by Almay, L'Oreal, Revlon, Maybelline, Mary Kay and Victoria Jackson.

Blush: In order for a blush to be good, it should be matte or have minimal shine and it should go on smoothly and easily. I'm glad to say I found plenty that qualify. I also found that it makes no sense to spend a lot of money on blushers. Many of the products at the drugstore are of a superior quality and provide the same results as those you will find at the department store. I particularly liked many of the new cream-to-powder blushers that I tried. These are a wonderful new type of blush that provides a very sheer, controlled application.

The best blushes are Adrien Arpel's Powdery Creme Blush, Almay's Cheek Color Blush, Cream-to-Powder Blush and Brush-On Blush, Borghese's Liquid Powder Blush and Regular Blush (only those shades that aren't shiny), Chanel's (only those shades that aren't shiny), Charles of the Ritz's, Christian Dior's, Clinique's Soft Pressed Powder Blush, Cover Girl's (all types, although the fragrance can be overpowering), Elizabeth Arden's, Estee Lauder's Soft Color Creme Blush and Signature Powder Blush (only those that aren't shiny), Lancome's Blush Majeur and Maquiriche, L'Oreal's Visuelle Powder Blush and Micro Blush, Mary Kay's Powder Perfect Cheek Color (powders only), Maybelline's Brush Blush, Origins', Revlon's Color Cling Blush (department store), Revlon's Glamorous Blush-On, Powder Creme Blush and Sheer Face Color (drugstore), Shiseido's, Ultima II's Creamy Powder Blush (only those shades that aren't shiny) and Victoria Jackson's.

The best buys without sacrificing quality are made by Almay, Charles of the Ritz, Clinique, Cover Girl, L'Oreal, and Revlon (both drugstore and department store).

Eyeshadow: As you already know, I can't tolerate shiny eyeshadows. As a result, I spent a great deal of time searching for the best of the matte shades—and I found them. I should mention that this wasn't an easy task because the preponderance of eyeshadows at both department stores and drugstores are mostly shiny. I've noticed that many of the lines are now introducing matte shades. As more consumers start to buy them, shiny eyeshadows will slowly but surely become much less dominant.

Be aware that all of the lines I'm listing here have some shiny eyeshadows mixed in with their matte colors. Please avoid the shiny ones at all costs. The best matte eyeshadows are: Charles of the Ritz's, Max Factor's Picture Perfect Eyeshadows (non-shiny only), Maybelline's (non-shiny only), Origins', Prescriptives', Revlon's Color Cling Eyeshadows (department store, non-shiny only) and Ultima II's New Nakeds. The best buys for matte eyeshadows are definitely at the drugstore.

Maybelline and Revlon have the most selections, but that isn't saying much. The department store cosmetics counters are where you can find the largest assortment of matte shades. The best selections are found at Charles of the Ritz, Origins, Prescriptives, and Ultima II.

Lipstick: There are some remarkable lipsticks on the market and I have found several that are unquestionably superior and more than reasonably priced. The best lipsticks are Adrien Arpel's Cream Lipstick, Almay's, Chanel's Rouge a Levres, Charles of the Ritz's Moisture Wear Lipstick, Christian Dior's, Clinique's Different Lipstick, Super Lipstick and Remoisturizing Lipstick, Cover Girl's Continuous Color, Elizabeth Arden's Luxury Lipstick, Estee Lauder's Perfect Lipstick and All Day Lipstick, Lancome's Hydra-Riche and Rouge Superb, L'Oreal's Colour Supreme, Creme Riche and L'Artiste Creme, Max Factor's Moisture Rich Lipstick, New Definition, Lasting Color Lipstick and Maxi's Soft Lustre Long Lasting Color, Maybelline's Long Wearing Lipstick, Prescriptives' Classic Lipstick, Revlon's Super Lustrous Creme, Moon Drops Moisture Creme and Moon Drop Luminesque (drugstore only) and Ultima II's Mattes, Lip Chrome and Super Luscious Lipstick.

The best buys and some of my absolute favorite lipsticks are from L'Oreal, Max Factor and Revlon (drugstore).

How to prevent lipstick from feathering into the lines around the mouth is of interest to many women, including myself. I was thrilled when I discovered Chanel's Protective Colour Control stick. It was one of the first products I've used that ever really kept my lipstick from bleeding. Imagine my excitement when I found a product by Coty called Stop-It ($4.50). It worked just as well as Chanel's, for one-third the price. Then I found Revlon's Color-Lock and that worked equally well for about the same price as Coty's Stop-It. (The only drawback for Revlon's Color-Lock is that it goes on slightly white, which will make your shade of lip color look lighter.) All these products have changed my life, because now I don't have to worry about accentuating the lines around my mouth every time I apply lipstick.

Lip Pencil: There is no reason to spend more than a few dollars on lip pencils. I can say without any hesitation that lip pencils priced over $6.00 are a waste of money. There is little to no difference between a higher priced pencil and a less expensive one. You can spend $22 on Estee Lauder's very attractive retractable lip pencil in the metallic blue case or you can spend $3 on Almay's or Revlon's (drug store) lip pencils and get the same look. The decision is up to you. The only real difference between pencils is that a few are more greasy than others. I recommend staying away from the greasy variety because they can smear and may not last as long as ones that are a bit drier.

The best lip pencils on the market, regardless of price are from Adrien Arpel, Almay, The Body Shop, Borghese, Chanel, Clinique, Cover Girl, Elizabeth Arden, Estee Lauder, Fashion Fair, Lancome, Mary Kay, Max Factor Lip Definer, Origin, Prescriptives, Revlon (drugstore) Waterproof Lip Shaper, Shiseido and Victoria Jackson.

Because lip pencils have so much in common, almost every line sells a good, reliable one. Price, therefore, become the most important criterion. The best buys are: Almay's, The Body Shop, Clinique's, Cover Girl's, Mary Kay's, Max Factor's, Revlon's (drugstore) and Victoria Jackson's.

Note: *Lip pencils do not stop lipstick from bleeding. They can slow it down a little, but that's about it. Lip liner shapes the mouth before you apply lipstick. Personally, I never have time for lip liner and I like the shape of my mouth, so I skip to the chase and use any of the anti-feathering products I mentioned above with my lipstick color.*

Eye Pencil: Most eye pencils have a lot of similarities, although there are definitely pencils on the market that are greasier than others. Whether eye pencils have a greasier or drier texture they can all cause problems. An eye pencil with a dry texture makes it difficult to line the eyelid after you've applied your eyeshadows; or if the pencil is more on the greasy side, it will line the lid more easily, but it is also more likely to smear under the lower lashes in a very short period of time. If you've read my book *Blue Eyeshadow Should Still Be Illegal* then you know that I prefer lining the eyes with regular eyeshadow powder and a small, thin eyeliner brush. I usually line my lower lashes with a soft brown eyeshadow and my eyelid with a black or dark brown eyeshadow. You can also wet the brush and apply the eyeshadow as you would a liquid liner in a more vivid line. In fact, even on the occasion that I line my eyes with a pencil, I go over it with an eyeshadow to make sure it stays all day. The difference of that look, and how long it lasts, in comparison to when you use a pencil alone, is amazing — particularly if you have oily or combination skin. If, however, the technique of lining your eyes with an eyeshadow and a tiny brush has eluded you and you still prefer pencils, then there are many companies that have good products. You can shop the more expensive lines, but it is simply a waste of money. At all price levels, I found many more similarities among pencils than differences.

The best eye pencils are Adrien Arpel's, Almay's (although the color selection is limited), Borghese's, Chanel's (only those that aren't iridescent), Charles of the Ritz's, Clinique's, Cover Girl's, Elizabeth Arden's, Estee Lauder's, Lancome's, L'Oreal's, Mary Kay's, Max Factor's Featherblend Kohliner, Maybelline's Expert Eyes Pencil, Origins', Revlon's Micropure Slimliner (drugstore), Shiseido's and Victoria Jackson's. The best buys and quality are without question from Almay, Charles of the Ritz, L'Oreal, Mary Kay, Max Factor, Origins, Revlon (drugstore) and Victoria Jackson. I also like Shiseido's pencils very much, but they are not exactly what I would call a bargain.

Almost every cosmetics line has a selection of liquid eyeliners. They vary from a traditional tube liner to a felt-tip type liner. Although I don't like the look a liquid liner provides, I understand that it is an option some women choose. In those situations, you will find the best liquid liners are found at Elizabeth Arden, Lancome, Max Factor, Maybelline and Revlon (drug store).

Eyebrow Pencil: Eyebrow pencil has long been the standard method for making eyebrows appear thicker or more defined. Most eyebrow pencils are identical to eyeliner pencils. Many companies sell only one type of pencil with appropriate colors for the brow. I have excluded all eyebrow pencils that are too greasy and can make the brow look "penciled." For a while, eyebrow powders were widely sold as an alternative to pencils. These brow powders were simply eyeshadows packaged under a different name. Only a handful of cosmetics companies still sell brow powders. This is not a reflection of how well they worked — eyebrow powders are an excellent, less obvious alternative to pencils, but it remains difficult for women to adopt this mode of filling in the eyebrow. Now there are several companies that make eyebrow gels. For the most part, these are great. I strongly recommend them as another way to make eyebrows look fuller but not artificial. If you can learn how to use the eyebrow gels, they can be a great alternative from pencils.

The best eyebrow pencils are from Adrien Arpel, Almay, Charles of the Ritz, Christian Dior (although the color selection is limited), Lancome and Shiseido.

The best eyebrow powders (which I prefer over brow pencils) are Elizabeth Arden's Brow Powders and Max Factor's Brush & Brow.

The best eyebrow gels are Borghese's (although the color selection is limited), Charles of the Ritz's Brow Definer and Visage's Brow Gel (the largest color selection of brow gels available, $15.50 each). Charles of the Ritz's version is by far my favorite for price and ease of application without having the brow getting thick and clumpy from the gel.

Note: *Visage is a cosmetic line that is available in better department stores. This line specializes in the custom blending of several makeup items, from lipsticks to eyeshadows to blushers. I did not include this line in my review because the results of the custom blending are totally dependent on the skill of the salesperson which, as you may already suspect, varied broadly counter to counter. Because of that variation, there was no way to review what you personally might receive.*

Mascara: I was quite surprised how many good mascaras there are at both drugstores and departments store. All price ranges include excellent mascaras. Obviously, I think it is foolish to buy the most expensive when the reasonably priced mascaras are equally as good, but again, the decision is up to you.

The best mascaras are Almay's One Coat Mascara and Mascara Plus, Chanel's Luxury Creme Mascara, Clinique's Supermascara, Estee Lauder's More Than Mascara, Lancome's, L'Oreal's Formula Riche and Lash Out Mascara, Max Factor's 2000 Calorie Mascara, Maybelline's Great Lash Mascara and No Problem Mascara, Prescriptives', Revlon's Long Distance Mascara and Quick Thick Mascara and Victoria Jackson's.

The best buys (and some of my favorites) are by Almay, L'Oreal, Max Factor, Maybelline, Revlon and Victoria Jackson.

Note: *Maybelline's Great Lash Mascara can have a slight tendency to smudge, particularly on oily skin types.*

Brushes: You would think basic necessities like the tools used to apply makeup would be readily available at cosmetics counters, but that is not the case. The choices are very limited. Lancome sells a nice selection of brushes, but they are expensive. There are two sizes of blush brushes available from Revlon and Cover Girl that are very good, but they can't be used to apply eyeshadows. Several department stores across the country sell an excellent, reasonably priced line of makeup brushes by Joan Simmons. If you can find them, they can handle the job nicely. My last suggestion, at least when it comes to tools for applying eyeshadows, is to try an art supply store. They have a vast selection of brushes in all price ranges that are perfect for sensitive lids.

Cleanser: I predicted almost a decade ago that most cosmetics companies would eventually offer a wide selection of water-soluble cleansers to the consumer. I believed that women were tired of wiping off their makeup every night. Pulling at the skin, tugging on delicate eyelashes, or washing with a bar soap that dries out the skin and burns the eyes were not great skin care options. Ten years later, I've been proved right. Now there is a vast selection of water-soluble cleansers on the market that clean the face and remove makeup. The only drawback to this success is that most of these formulas are either too drying, too greasy or uneffective. More often than not the cleansers I tested that claimed to be water-soluble were actually meant to be wiped off with a washcloth instead of a tissue. Well, a washcloth is better than tissue, but only slightly; rubbing and pulling at the face is not good for the skin no matter how you do it. The ideal cleanser should rinse off easily with gentle splashing and neither dry the skin or leave a greasy residue.

The other type of water-soluble cleansers I found on the market contained ingredients that had more in common with shampoos than they did anything else. These were definitely great at cleaning the face, but they almost all left a very dry feeling behind on the skin and often caused irritation around the eye area. These kind of sudsing or foaming water-soluble cleansers are often recommended for women with oily or combination skin types. In my opinion it doesn't make sense for any skin type, more or less someone with oily skin, to dry out their skin with any product. Using a drying cleanser inevitably will require the use of a moisturizer. Moisturizers are almost always a problem for someone with oily or combination skin. Besides, this cycle of drying out oily or combination skin and then following up with a moisturizer is the fastest way I know to cause skin problems.

Does it make sense to spend a lot of money on a cleanser? As it turns out the cleansers I liked best were also the least expensive. Believe me, I wanted to find other cleansers to recommend. I even disregarded price categories in the beginning of my research so I could remain as impartial as possible — but there just weren't many cleansers out there that met my qualifications. After an exhaustive search the best water-soluble cleansers I found that really cleansed the face, removed eye makeup and didn't dry the skin or leave it feeling greasy were Neutrogena's Facial Cleansing Formula, Revlon's Clean & Clear Facial Cleansing Gel and Clean & Clear Facial Cleansing Gel for Sensitive Skin and Owen/Galderma's Cetaphil Lotion. These were also the best buys.

Scrub Products: Scrub products are a primary way to help exfoliate (slough off) dead skin cells which is an important part of most skin care routines. The problems occur when you use either a drying cleanser or a drying toner and then a facial scrub or all three, or, even worse a facial scrub that is too irritating and too abrasive. Too much exfoliating can be bad for the skin. I suggest using either a gentle toner (see next section) or a scrub, but definitely not both and never one right after the other. Personally, I recommend using baking soda mixed with water as a way to exfoliate the skin instead of the scrubs you can buy on the market. I prefer it to every other scrub or exfoliating cleanser I tested. Generally, I only recommend 3% hydrogen peroxide in place of a toner for those women who have a problem with blackheads or acne. (See Chapter Four for more detailed skin care information.)

Toner: By now you are probably well aware that I would never recommend a product for the face that contained alcohol or any irritating ingredients. Toners and all the products that fall into this category (refining lotions, clarifying lotions, soothing tonics, stimulating lotions, fresheners and astringents) are an extra cleansing step that have been around so long it is hard for most women to imagine doing without it. You are supposed to be believe that these products can do everything from refresh the skin to close pores to exfoliate the skin, or simply clean the face that one extra time. Of all the claims toners boast, the only thing toners can do is clean the face and exfoliate the skin. If they didn't contain irritating ingredients, they could also soothe the skin and leave it feeling moist. I evaluated these products strictly on how soothing and clean they felt on the face without drying the skin or leaving a greasy residue.

Does it make sense to spend a lot of money on a toner if it doesn't contain irritating ingredients? No, I found excellent toners that had very gentle ingredients and were relatively inexpensive. For those women who enjoy using these products, and because of the soothing, fresh feeling many irritant-free toners can provide, I feel they can be beneficial for many skin types. The best ones are Adrien Arpel's Herbal Astringent, The Body Shop's Orange Flower Water and Honey Water, Borghese's Tonico Minerale, Chanel's Lotion Douce, Christian Dior's Skin Freshener, Clinique's Alcohol-Free Clarifier, Estee Lauder's Gentle Protection Tonic and Re-Nutriv Gentle Skin Toner, La Prairie's Cellular Purifying Lotion, Lancome's Tonique Douceur, L'Oreal's Floral Tonic, Mary Kay's Gentle Action Freshener, Physicians Formula Gentle Refreshing Toner, Ultima II's CHR Extraordinary Gentle Clarifier and Victoria Jackson's Toning Mist.

The best buys are found at The Body Shop, Clinique, L'Oreal, Mary Kay, Physicians Formula, Ultima II and Victoria Jackson.

Moisturizer: I'm including in this category all lotions, creams, wrinkle creams, specialty creams and lotions that are designed to eliminate dry skin. Surprisingly enough, I liked almost all the moisturizers I reviewed. Even wrinkle creams — which won't get rid of wrinkles — almost all contained ingredients that make them good moisturizers. Of course, I intensely dislike the exaggerated claims that accompany these products, but that shouldn't be the least bit surprising to you by now. Only a handful of moisturizers contained ingredients that I thought were potentially harmful to the skin. Other than that, there are really some remarkable products on the market, in all price categories, containing great ingredients that can take care of varying degrees of dry skin.

When it comes to moisturizers, the problem for most women is finding a moisturizer that is the right one for their skin type. Some moisturizers contain extremely rich ingredients such as lanolin, vegetable oil, mineral oil, petrolatum, shea butter, cocoa butter or protein that are best for only those women with very dry skin. Then there are various forms of lighter weight moisturizers that contain only one or two oils and these are best for skin that is normal to dry. If you do not have extremely dry skin stay away from moisturizers that are loaded with the ingredients I mentioned above. If you have slightly or occasionally dry skin you are better off with those moisturizers that contain only one or two oils. Finding the appropriate type of moisturizer for your skin will be easier if you review the ingredients I've listed for the moisturizers in Chapter Seven.

All dry skin can gain benefit to some degree from moisturizing ingredients such as sodium pca, hyaluronic acid, collagen, elastin, retinyl palmitate and vitamin E. The other "specialty" ingredients such as cow extract, spleen extract, tissue extract, placental extract, serum protein, mineral salts, flower or plant extracts can be completely ignored or avoided altogether.

If you are wondering about day cream versus night creams my recommendation is to ignore those categories of products and go by what your skin needs. If your skin is extremely dry, products rich in oils and lanolin may be necessary for your skin morning and night. If you have skin that is dry, but not excessively so, you may want to use a light moisturizing lotion that contains one or two oils in the morning and a more emollient cream at night. If you have slightly dry skin, a lightweight moisturizer should be perfect for both morning and night. Do you need an eye or throat cream? I know this sounds completely contrary to everything you've heard or read about skin care, but no you do not need a special eye or throat cream. The moisturizer you use on your face will work around your eyes. Try to disregard the scare tactics you hear at the cosmetics counters, or the brochures you read that carry on about special formulations designed exclusively for the eye area. These claims are not substantiated by the ingredients in the product which are practically identical when compared to a cream supposedly designed just for the face.

For those women with oily skin, my strong suggestion, is to not get sucked into believing that oily skin needs a moisturizer to prevent the skin from wrinkling. Unless we are talking about a sunscreen with an SPF of 15 or greater, there are no moisturizers on the market that will do more for you skin than your own oil can do. The oil on your face is your own built in moisturizer. Moisturizers on the market are all trying to duplicate what the oil in your skin is supposed to be naturally doing for you. If you have oily skin that is also dry read over Chapter Four before you decide to go shopping for a moisturizer.

Does it make sense to spend a lot of money on moisturizers? Now after you've read this whole book, you tell me. The best moisturizers on the market for extremely dry skin are to be found at every skin care line on the market! Please read the particular information under each skin care line in Chapter Seven to evaluate the particular product you are considering and get used to reading skin care ingredients. The best buys, however, are to be found at Almay, The Body Shop, Eucerin, L'Oreal, Lubriderm, Mary Kay, Neutrogena, Nivea, Nutraderm, Oil of Olay, Physicians Formula, Pond's, Revlon (both drugstore and department store) and Victoria Jackson.

Specialty Products: Although I am rarely a woman of few words, I feel quite comfortable stating that there were no specialty products (such as facial masks or skin treatments) on the market that I thought were particularly exceptional for the skin or worth the exceptional price tag.

"The question is not, can they reason?
Nor, can they talk?
But, can they suffer?"

CHAPTER NINE

Beauty That Respects Nature

CRUELTY FREE MAKEUP

"Natural" products, to me, are products that have not been tested on animals. To deform and kill animal life in futile, inconclusive and absurdly cruel tests in the name of safety are "unnatural" and inhumane. I should explain that I am not an expert on the subject of animal-free testing nor do I want to create the illusion that I am. However, I do support many knowledgeable groups who are active both politically and socially in changing common animal testing practices that they feel (and, from everything I've read about both sides of the issue, I concur) have no relevancy on how a product will effect a person's skin or health. I find the research information these groups have available both disturbing and poignant. My sources of information are: **National Anti-Vivisection Society**, 53 West Jackson Boulevard, Chicago, Illinois, 60604, (312) 427-6065, and **People for the Ethical Treatment of Animals (PETA)**, P.O. Box 42516, Washington, D.C. 20015, (301) 770-7444. The basic philosophy of both groups is as long as there are thousands of cruelty-free products available that are safe and effective, and as long as there are reliable means of testing without using animals, there is no excuse for the continued use of tests that torture animal life. For more details about animal-free testing alternatives, please write to these organizations.

It is important to explain that the following lists do not reflect in any way the quality of the products the companies produce. Companies in each list sell products that can be either wonderful or a complete waste of money.

This first list is simply a compilation of cosmetics companies that do not test or contract anyone to test their products on animals. I respect the responsible and humane position these businesses have chosen to follow. I applaud their lead in this controversial issue. It is through their efforts that we move closer to achieving a more caring and compassionate world. The names of the companies listed below were taken from the booklet *Personal Care with Principles,* published by the National Anti-Vivisection Society. For a complete list of such companies (not just those involved with cosmetics), I recommend that you write and request a copy of this booklet.

The following cosmetics companies do not use animal testing:
Adrien Arpel
Alexandra de Markoff (Revlon)
Almay (Revlon)
Amway
Aramis (Estee Lauder)
Aveda
Avon
Beauty Without Cruelty (England)
Beiersdorf
Bill Blass (Revlon)
The Body Shop
Bonnie Bell
Charles of the Ritz (Revlon)
Christian Dior Perfumes
Clarins
Clinique (Estee Lauder)
Color Me Beautiful
Crabtree & Evelyn
Estee Lauder
Fashion Two Twenty
Germaine Monteil (Revlon)
Guerlain
Halston (Revlon)
I Natural Cosmetics
Ida Grae Cosmetics
Jergens
Lubriderm

Mary Kay Cosmetics (they have just established a moratorium on animal
    testing; they may return to it without notice)
Max Factor (Revlon)
Merle Norman Cosmetics
Natural Wonder (Revlon)
Nexxus Products
Nivea
Nu Skin International
Paul Mitchell Systems
Prescriptives (Estee Lauder)
Rachel Perry
Redken Labs
Revlon
Sebastian International
Shaklee U.S.
St. Ives Labs
Ultima II (Revlon)
Visage Beaute Cosmetics
Warner-Lambert Company

The following cosmetics companies continue to use animal testing:
Alberto Culver
Bain de Soleil
Breck
Bristol-Meyers
Camay
Chanel
Chesebrough-Pond's
Clairol
Clarion
Clearasil
Coty
Cover Girl
Cutex
Dermassage
Dove
Elizabeth Arden
Erno Lazlo
Georgette Klinger

Helena Rubenstein
Ivory
Johnson & Johnson
Lancome
L'Oreal
Maybelline
Neutrogena Skincare Institute
Nina Ricci
Noxell
Oil of Olay
Paloma Picasso
Pantene
Physicians Formula (this company, which had recently eliminated testing their products on animals, has been purchased by a manufacturer that uses animal testing)
Pond's
Proctor & Gamble
Ralph Lauren Products
Vidal Sassoon Products
Yves St. Laurent Products

Index

ABOUT THE AUTHOR

PAULA BEGOUN began her career as a makeup artist more than 12 years ago, in Washington D.C. From there she moved to Seattle, Washington, where she opened a chain of cosmetics stores called Generic Makeup. These stores were unique because they sold only one skin care product. The other components of Paula's skin care regimen were products obtainable at the drugstore or the grocery store. During that time Paula also appeared as a feature reporter on the Noon News at KIRO-TV and KIRO-Radio in Seattle. As rewarding as she found her work in the media, Paula felt she was really an entrepreneur at heart and decided to try other avenues of self-employment. She sold her makeup stores, left broadcasting in 1985 and started her own publishing company.

Paula's first book *Blue Eyeshadow Should be Illegal* and the revised, updated edition *Blue Eyeshadow Should STILL Be Illegal — The World After Retin-A: What Do You Do Now?* were best-sellers in the U.S., Canada and Australia. Having appeared on countless talk shows, including Oprah Winfrey, Phil Donahue, Sally Jesse Raphael and the CBS Morning News, she continues to make a difference in the way women view the cosmetics industry by providing forthright evaluations and alternative solutions. With humor and straightforward information about cosmetics, Retin-A, and a dozen other beauty-related topics, Paula continues to educate and influence consumer-minded women.